ULTRA-WIDE FIELD PHOTOGRAPHY ATLAS OF
RETINOPATHY OF PREMATURITY

ULTRA-WIDE FIELD PHOTOGRAPHY ATLAS OF
RETINOPATHY OF PREMATURITY

Sushma Ratna Jayanna MBBS DNB FICO
Vitreo-Retina Surgeon and Faculty In-charge of ROP Services
Shantilal Shanghvi Eye Institute
Mumbai, Maharashtra, India
(Former Fellow and Faculty, LV Prasad Eye Institute, Hyderabad)

Foreword
Subhadra Jalali

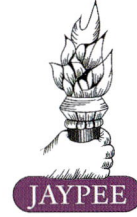

JAYPEE BROTHERS MEDICAL PUBLISHERS
The Health Sciences Publisher
New Delhi | London

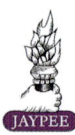

Jaypee Brothers Medical Publishers (P) Ltd

Headquarters
Jaypee Brothers Medical Publishers (P) Ltd
EMCA House, 23/23-B
Ansari Road, Daryaganj
New Delhi 110 002, India
Landline: +91-11-23272143, +91-11-23272703
+91-11-23282021, +91-11-23245672
Email: jaypee@jaypeebrothers.com

Corporate Office
Jaypee Brothers Medical Publishers (P) Ltd
4838/24, Ansari Road, Daryaganj
New Delhi 110 002, India
Phone: +91-11-43574357
Fax: +91-11-43574314
Email: jaypee@jaypeebrothers.com

Overseas Office
JP Medical Ltd.
83, Victoria Street, London
SW1H 0HW (UK)
Phone: +44 20 3170 8910
Fax: +44 (0)20 3008 6180
Email: info@jpmedpub.com

Website: www.jaypeebrothers.com
Website: www.jaypeedigital.com

© 2024, Jaypee Brothers Medical Publishers

The views and opinions expressed in this book are solely those of the original contributor(s)/author(s) and do not necessarily represent those of editor(s) or publisher of the book.

All rights reserved. No part of this publication may be reproduced, stored or transmitted in any form or by any means, electronic, mechanical, photocopying, recording or otherwise, without the prior permission in writing of the publishers.

All brand names and product names used in this book are trade names, service marks, trademarks or registered trademarks of their respective owners. The publisher is not associated with any product or vendor mentioned in this book.

Medical knowledge and practice change constantly. This book is designed to provide accurate, authoritative information about the subject matter in question. However, readers are advised to check the most current information available on procedures included and check information from the manufacturer of each product to be administered, to verify the recommended dose, formula, method and duration of administration, adverse effects and contraindications. It is the responsibility of the practitioner to take all appropriate safety precautions. Neither the publisher nor the author(s)/editor(s) assume any liability for any injury and/or damage to persons or property arising from or related to use of material in this book.

This book is sold on the understanding that the publisher is not engaged in providing professional medical services. If such advice or services are required, the services of a competent medical professional should be sought.

Every effort has been made where necessary to contact holders of copyright to obtain permission to reproduce copyright material. If any have been inadvertently overlooked, the publisher will be pleased to make the necessary arrangements at the first opportunity.

Inquiries for bulk sales may be solicited at: jaypee@jaypeebrothers.com

Ultra-Wide Field Photography Atlas of Retinopathy of Prematurity

First Edition: **2024**

ISBN: 978-93-5696-949-0

Printed at: Samrat Offset Pvt. Ltd.

Dedicated to

Dr Subhadra Jalali
A remarkable pediatric retina surgeon, an exceptional clinician,
and an affectionate mentor

Foreword

"*Sarvendriyanam Nayanam Pradhanam*"—the eyes are the most important of all the sense organs. In more than 30 years of my work as a "Retina" Specialist, I am amazed how little is known about this beautiful essential organ inside the depth of our eyes, where "Vision" is generated so that one can see!

Being hidden from sight, the "Retina" has been a difficult tissue to relate to by not only the students of various branches of medicine but even those training in eye diseases—the Ophthalmologists. Given that changes visible in the retina are known to reflect various disease conditions of the human body, every medical student needs to know about a normal and an abnormal retina. The problem becomes even more critical, when one tries to explain retinal problems to patients and relatives as they have no clue about the silent "Retina" which has no pain fibers and no external eye signs once it starts to suffer a disease. When it comes to the retina of newborns and tiny premature babies, the problem obviously gets compounded significantly. It ultimately results in babies getting inadequate eye care and can result in permanent incurable childhood blindness.

What our Pediatric Retina Specialists and Optometrists at LV Prasad Eye Institute have ventured to do is to use the Optos wide field retinal imaging system to its full potential to photograph the retina of premature babies in the outpatient department and open this amazing tissue to the eyes of the world! The pictures in themselves highlight very well various aspects of retinopathy of prematurity (ROP), a potentially blinding retinal disorder seen in premature babies that starts soon after birth and needs medical attention within 2030 days of life.

Taking retinal pictures of babies is only one part; to compile them into a meaningful atlas is a different ball game that requires dedication, focus on details, a passion for preventing newborn blindness and many hours of hard work. Who better to take on this task than Dr Sushma Ratna Jayanna, who started off as a Retina Fellow in the department and went on to become a keen student of ROP, trying to learn the difficult techniques of retinal examination in tiny babies. She is now an Expert Teacher and Practitioner in this field.

The atlas compiled by her will be a great additional tool for students to understand what to look for and shorten their learning curve. At the same time, the atlas will be of immense help to communicate the problem to parents, nurses, neonatologists, pediatricians, and health-media communicators. The vividly captured retinal images are accompanied by text legends explaining the clinical context and interpretation. The atlas also highlights the technique of taking these images effectively and safely and the few artifacts one must be careful about while interpreting the images. It is an awesome piece of work created by the currently named Anant Bajaj Retina Institute Team at LV Prasad Eye Institute and curated so well by Dr Jayanna.

When the student excels the teacher, it becomes an exhilarating moment for the teacher and the institution. It is a great honor and pleasure to go through the atlas and pen down its foreword. I am sure that this ROP atlas will be an indispensable tool in the clinics of Eye Specialists and Child Specialists when it comes to the "VISION" of our newborn premature babies. My Best wishes to see this happen!

Subhadra Jalali
Network Director
Newborn Eye Health Alliance (NEHA)
LV Prasad Eye Institute Network
Hyderabad, Telangana, India

Preface

My fascination for retinopathy of prematurity (ROP) started during my early days of retina fellowship in the LV Prasad Eye Institute, Hyderabad, Telangana, India in the year 2018. The credit for inculcating the interest on such an elaborate disease, in young minds like mine goes to Dr Subhadra Jalali, who till today, keenly involves herself in treating the eyes of premature babies and training amateur surgeons with kindness and grace. When I was being intimidated by the complexities of adult retinal pathologies and surgeries in my initial days of training, here was an amazing surgeon teaching me, the most challenging subject of ROP in a most simplified way possible. If my interest in ROP has exponential growth till date, that will be majorly because of Dr Jalali. It is through her I have realized that the responsibility of a student's sheer involvement in any subject lies solely with the mentor who is wise enough to demystify any complex subject in a way that reaches out to mentees without appalling them. This atlas on ROP is fashioned in a similar view to make it comprehensible not only to ophthalmologist but also to reach out to pediatricians and neonatologists whose active involvement is crucial in the management of ROP. The atlas presents ultra-wide field photographs of various findings at different stages and types of ROP systematically along with a brief summary explaining the pathogenesis. These Images were captured by trained technicians in an everyday busy outpatient department with immense patience and diligence. Without their active involvement, this atlas was close to impossible. Handing over the first rough copy of this atlas to my mentor Dr Jalali as a parting gift after completing my tenure at LVPEI, Hyderabad in beginning of 2020 was one of the most gratifying moments in my professional life. I cannot be grateful enough to Dr Taraprasad Das, who has been a mentor to my mentor, for constantly motivating and guiding me to reach the finishing line of this atlas. I feel immensely blessed for having a chance to interact with such an exceptionally intellectual mind through the making of this atlas. I am deeply indebted to him for his help in shaping this book.

I hope this atlas helps Physicians, Ophthalmologists, Students, and Trainees across the world, in better comprehension of a complex disease like ROP to a significant extent.

Sushma Ratna Jayanna

Acknowledgments

OPHTHALMOLOGISTS

- Dr Abilasha Alone
- Dr Adnan Shaikh
- Dr Akash Belanje
- Dr Anirudh Soni
- Dr Avantika Dogra
- Dr Brijesh Takkar
- Dr Deepika CP
- Dr Destaw Muli
- Dr Deven Dhurandhar
- Dr Divya Balakrishnan
- Dr Hitesh Agrawal
- Dr Komal Agarwal
- Dr Niroj K Sahoo
- Dr Padmaja Kumari Rani
- Dr Renuka Chakurkar
- Dr Shashwath Behera
- Dr Subhadra Jalali
- Dr Virangi Doshi

OPTOMETRISTS

- Mr Agniv Dutta
- Mr Balaji Govindan
- Ms Kruthika Kannan
- Mr Kalmuri Mahesh
- Ms Neelima Manchikanti
- Mrs Preeti Pandey
- Ms Priya Jana
- Mr Seetaram Palavalasa
- Mr Srinivas Babburi
- Mr Subba Rao
- Mr Ugandhar Reddy

COMMUNICATIONS

- Mr Kishore Nookala
- Mrs Neha Hassija

Courtesy: All Images were taken from Optos Ultra-Wide Field Camera (Optos, Dunfermline, UK) at LV Prasad Eye Institute, Kallam Anji Reddy (KAR) Campus, Hyderabad, Telangana, India.

The Optos Daytona plus machine courtesy Cornell Medical Instruments (CMI), India.

Contents

1. Ultra-Wide Field Imaging Technique in Infants 1
2. Common Clinical Presentations in Retinopathy of Prematurity 7
3. Peculiar Findings in Retinopathy of Prematurity 22
4. Atypical Presentations of Retinopathy of Prematurity 34
5. Interventions and Follow-up in Retinopathy of Prematurity 39
6. Uncommon Associations in Retinopathy of Prematurity 59
7. Artifact in Ultra-Wide Field Photos 65

Index *69*

Abbreviations

A-ROP	:	Aggressive retinopathy of prematurity
APROP	:	Aggressive posterior retinopathy of prematurity
BIO	:	Binocular indirect ophthalmoscope
BW	:	Birth weight
GA	:	Gestational age
ICROP	:	International classification of retinopathy of prematurity
LIO	:	Laser indirect ophthalmoscopy
OD	:	Right eye
OPD	:	Outpatient department
OS	:	Left eye
OU	:	Both eyes
PMA	:	Postmenstrual age
ROP	:	Retinopathy of prematurity
UWF	:	Ultra-wide field
VEGF	:	Vascular endothelial growth factor

Ultra-Wide Field Imaging Technique in Infants

■ INTRODUCTION

The importance of documentation of fundus findings in retinopathy of prematurity (ROP) in today's era cannot be emphasized enough. It has proven to be a great tool for retinal specialists in the objective assessment of the findings, educating the trainees, and counseling of the parents.

A few of the commonly used fundus imaging modalities in ROP include RetCam (Clarity Medical Systems, Pleasanton, CA, USA) and Neo Forus (Bengaluru, India) with a limited field of imaging (130°). Ultra-wide field (UWF) photographs (Optos, Dunfermline, UK) which are mainly used for adult retinal pathologies, have been also tried in babies and have proven to be safe, efficient, and fast in everyday clinical practice. The significant advantage of UWF over other modalities is the noncontact camera and wider field of view (anteroposterior 200° field), which can be achieved in one capture. The confocal scanning laser ophthalmoscopy system in UWF cameras has less scattering of light and helps in obtaining a clearer image. An image size of 20 Mb can be captured in a quarter of a second. A special position, called the *flying baby* is adopted which is different from the conventional lying down position, to capture images using UWF cameras in babies under topical anesthesia.

It is at times challenging to image preterm infants as they usually will have systemic comorbidities and it is crucial to keep in mind the red flag signs, such as baby turning blue, change in tone of crying, sudden stoppage of cry, regurgitations and distension of abdomen, respiratory distress, feeding tubes, and apneic spells. Such babies need constant monitoring of vitals throughout the procedure and ideally, in order to have a standby pediatrician or a neonatal anesthetist.

This atlas comprises UWF photographs of various presentations and stages of ROP captured in an outpatient department (OPD) set-up of the LV Prasad Eye Institute, Hyderabad, India. All images were taken by trained technicians, on Optos UWF scanning laser ophthalmoscope camera Panoramic 200Tx imaging system (Optos PLC, Dunfermline, UK).

■ IMAGING TECHNIQUE

A written parental consent is obtained. A detailed history is taken in the OPD. Pupil dilatation is done using tropicamide (0.8%) and phenylephrine (2.5%) with instillation of one drop every 10 minutes for 30 minutes. Care must be taken to wipe out the excessive spillover of the drop to prevent systemic absorption through the skin.

Examination of the dilated fundus by the retinal specialist using a binocular indirect ophthalmoscope (BIO) and 20 diopter lens in a dimly lit room and grading of the disease is documented in the case sheet. Baby needs to be fed and burped at least half an hour before the procedure. The baby should be wrapped well with a warm clean cloth sheet, which helps in easy handling. Proparacaine 0.5% eye drops is used as a topical anesthetic agent, instilled before inserting a sterile pediatric lid speculum to retract the eyelids.

■ MODIFIED FLYING BABY POSITIONING

Technicians who are well versed in imaging adults and especially trained for 4–6 weeks, in handling preterm babies are involved. It requires a minimum of two of these technicians.

During the procedure, one arm of the trained technician supports the chest and the chin of the baby with the other hand supporting the head. Pupils are aligned by moving the head, with the movement of the eye guided by visual feedback on the monitor. After optimal positioning of the eye, images are captured by a second trained technician. The time taken for capturing the image after alignment is approximately 3 seconds. The Optos camera consists of a removable camera aperture of different sizes. A bigger aperture is used in small babies; a smaller aperture is used in bigger babies as it is easy to achieve alignment. In very tiny babies, eye alignment is easier without using any aperture, as the aperture could itself induce artifacts and shadowing.[1]

MODIFIED FLYING BABY TECHNIQUE

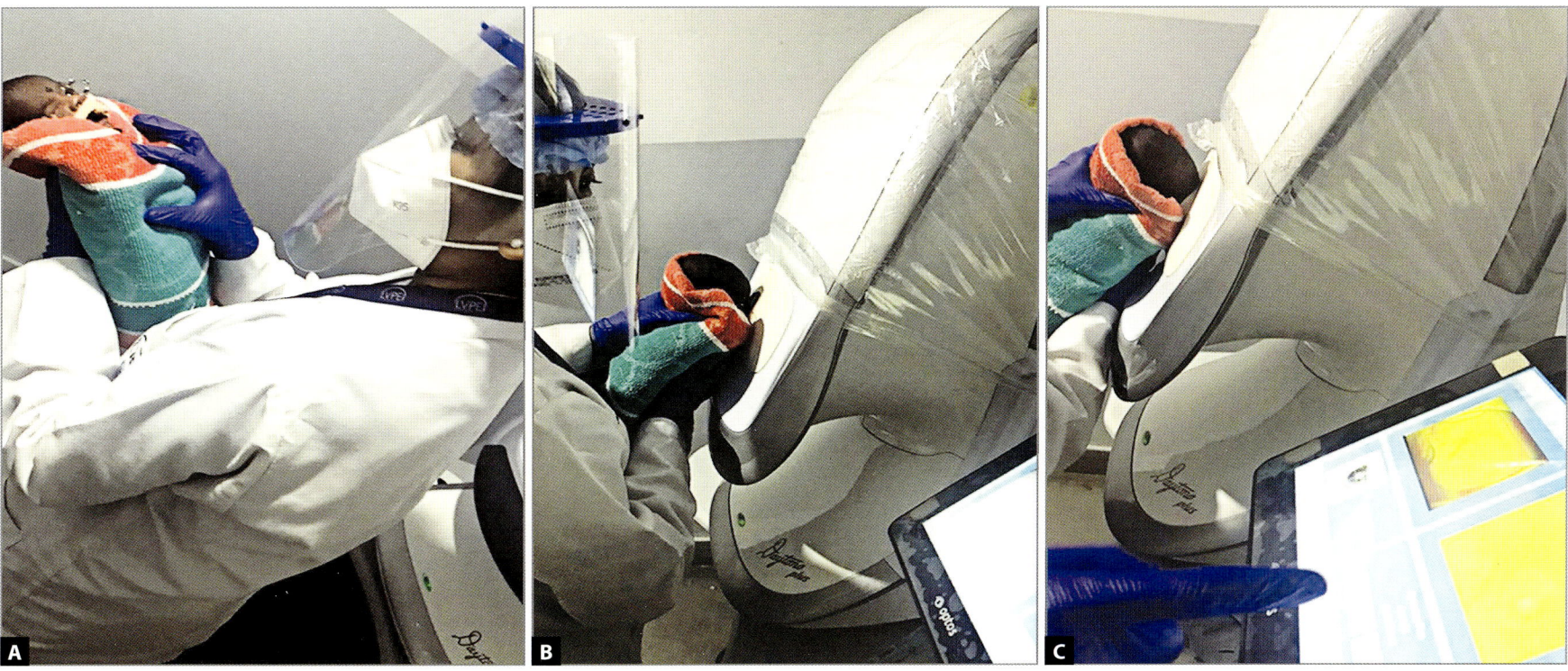

Figs. 1A to C: Modified flying baby positioning. (A) The baby is wrapped with warm clean clothes and a sterile speculum is inserted after topical anesthesia; (B) One arm of the technician supports the chest and the chin of the baby and the other hand supports the head. Pupils are aligned by moving the head, with the movement of the eye guided by visual feedback on the monitor; (C) After optimal positioning of the eye, images are then captured by a second trained technician.

■ MODIFICATION TO THE EXISTING APERTURES OF OPTOS

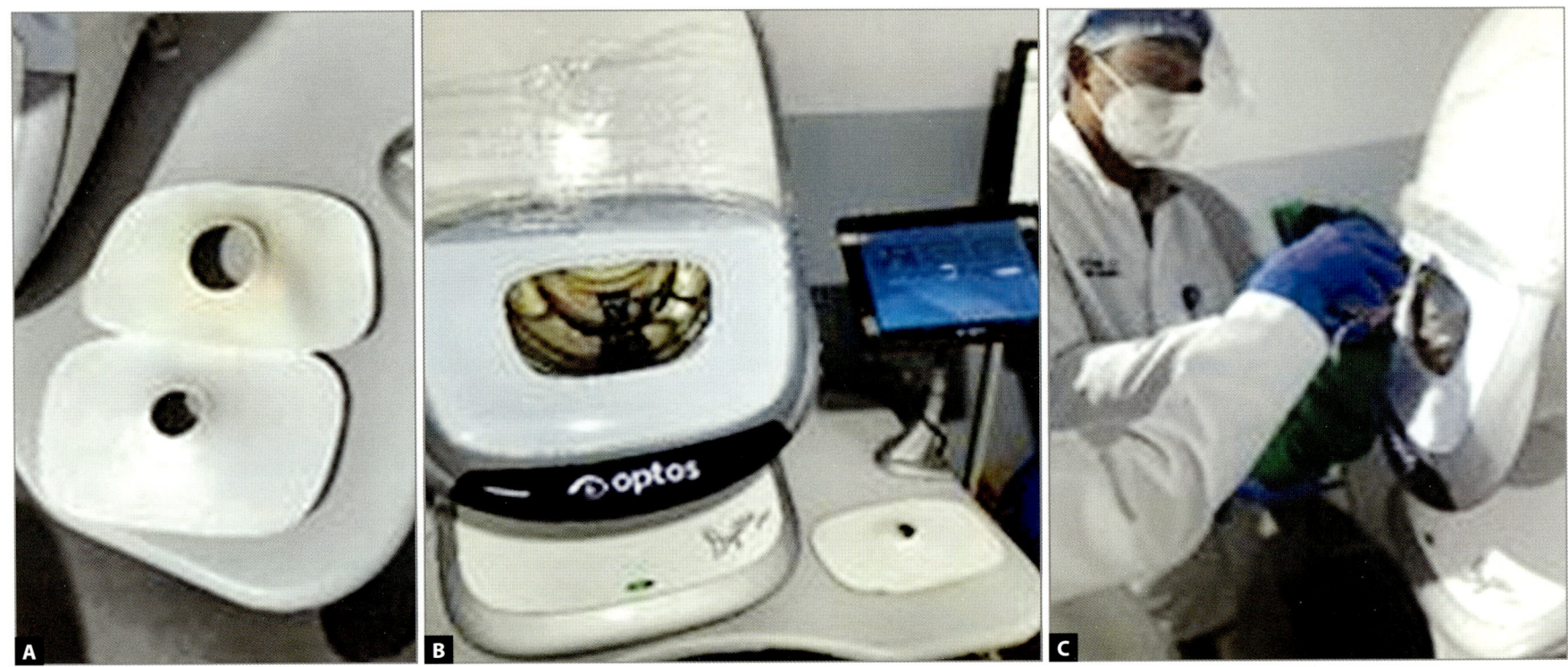

Figs. 2A to C: (A) Removable camera aperture of different sizes; (B) In very tiny babies, images are captured without using any aperture; (C) Aligning the pupil by moving the head with help of visual feedback monitor.

■ RETINA IN NEWBORN PRETERM BABY

Retinal vascularization starts in utero during 16 weeks of gestational age (GA) with vessels reaching the nasal side of the ora serrata by 36 weeks and the temporal side by 40 weeks, just before the birth of term baby. A mature retina in a newborn term baby appears completely vascularized with normal dichotomously branching vessels reaching up to the zone III anterior till the ora serrata.[2] Premature infants will have incompletely vascularized retina in the periphery, with either major retinal vessels in the affected zone or a complete avascular peripheral retina at birth.[2]

Both Eyes Mature Retina

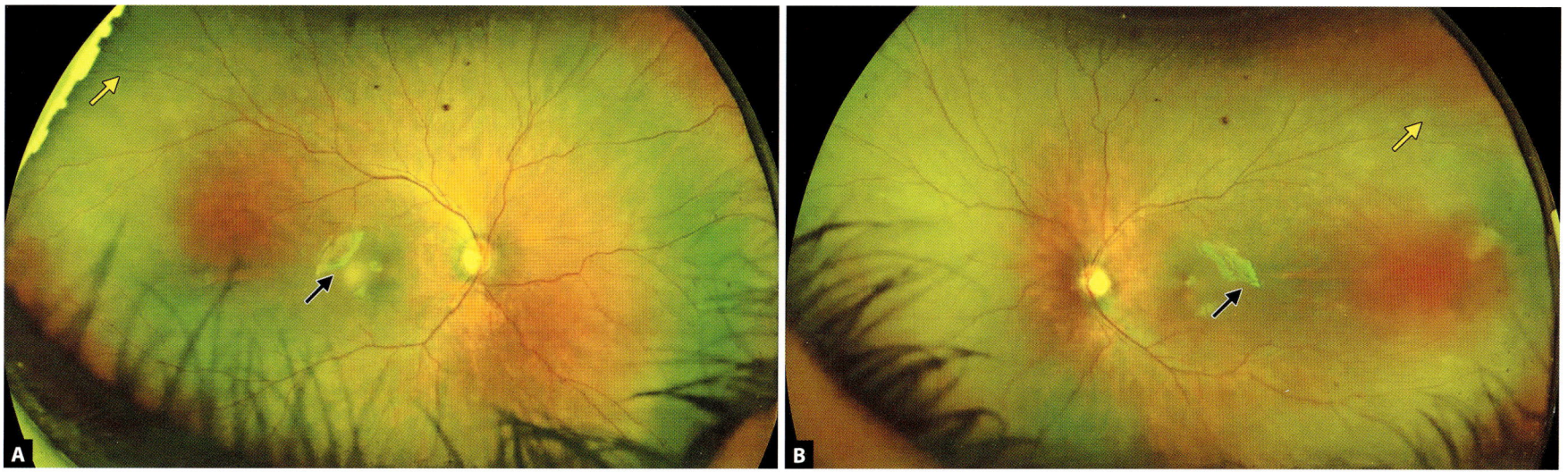

Figs. 3A and B: OU UWF fundus images of baby with 41 weeks postmenstrual age, 28 weeks gestational age and 2.5 kg birth weight with mature retina, normal dichotomously branching retinal vessels till zone III anterior (yellow arrows). Both the images show reflection artefact (black arrows). (OU: both eyes; UWF: ultra-wide field)

Both Eyes Immature Retina Zones II and III

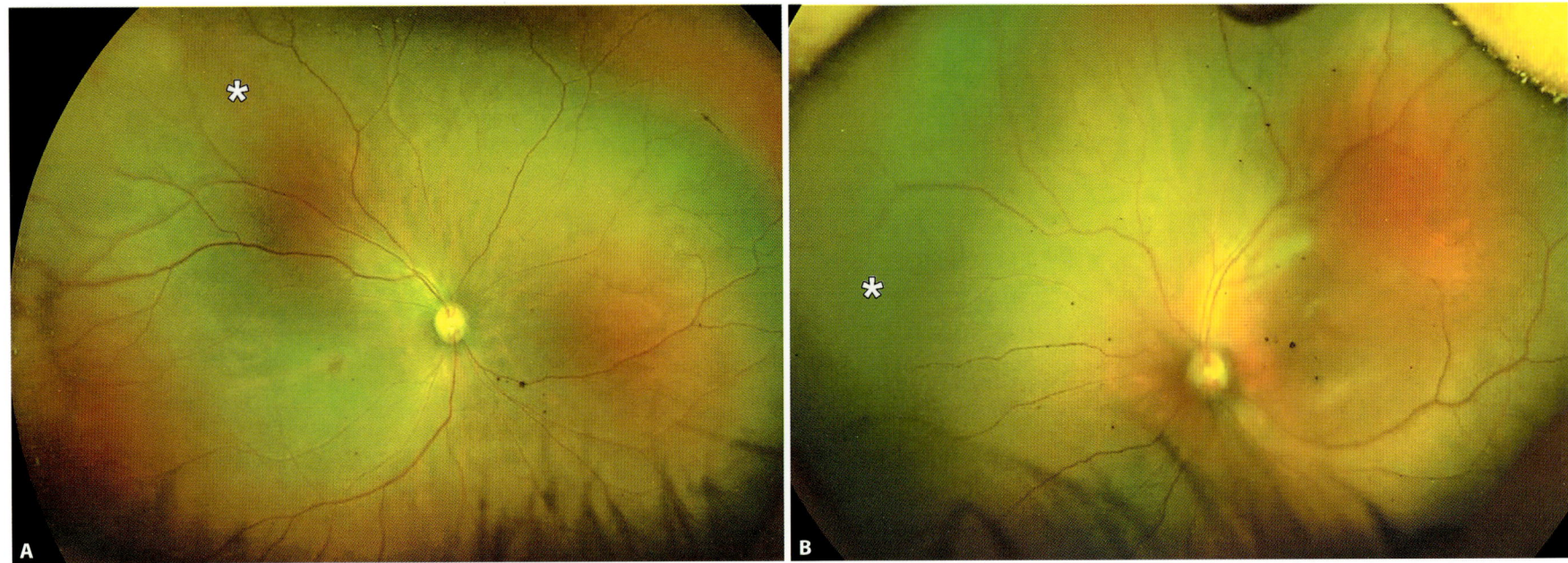

Figs. 4A and B: OU UWF fundus images of baby with 36 weeks PMA, 28 weeks GA and 900 g of BW showing immature retina (asterisks) with the presence of only major vessels in zones II and III. (BW: birth weight; GA: gestational age; OU: both eyes; PMA: postmenstrual age; UWF: ultra-wide field)

■ REFERENCES

1. Jayanna S, Agarwal K, Doshi V, Reddy RU, Ali H, Dogra A, et al. A retrospective analysis of ultra-widefield photograph (Optos) documentation of retinopathy of prematurity at a tertiary eye care outpatient setup: the Indian Twin Cities ROP Study, report number 11. J AAPOS. 2022;26(2):68.e1-6.
2. Sun Y, Smith LEH. Retinal vasculature in development and diseases [retracted in: Annu Rev Vis Sci. 2020;15;0:10.]. Annu Rev Vis Sci. 2018;4:101-22.

Common Clinical Presentations in Retinopathy of Prematurity

■ INTRODUCTION

Retinopathy of prematurity (ROP) is one of the significant concern in neonatal care, as it can lead to irreversible blindness in preterm babies. For a clinician to diagnose and manage this condition, understanding its common clinical features becomes crucial. This chapter provides a comprehensive roadmap to recognize and assess the various common clinical presentations.

■ AGGRESSIVE RETINOPATHY OF PREMATURITY

Aggressive retinopathy of prematurity (A-ROP) or earlier called aggressive posterior retinopathy of prematurity (APROP) is a rapidly progressive form of ROP. It manifests with retinal neovascularization, extensive tortuosity, and looping of blood vessels; it usually involves the posterior pole but can extend beyond it.[1] Important risk factor for the development of A-ROP is attributed to a disruption in vasculogenesis due to various factors including extreme prematurity, low platelet count, supplementation of unblended oxygen, and sepsis.[2,3] Though, it was initially thought to be occurring in extremely tiny babies, [<30 weeks gestational age (GA), <1,000 g birth weight (BW)] recent studies have shown that it can also occur in older and heavier preterm babies of BW >1,500 g. Such babies usually present with flat new vessels in posterior zone II with large vessels looping with preserved posterior arcade vessels.[3]

■ BOTH EYES AGGRESSIVE RETINOPATHY OF PREMATURITY (Scenario 1)

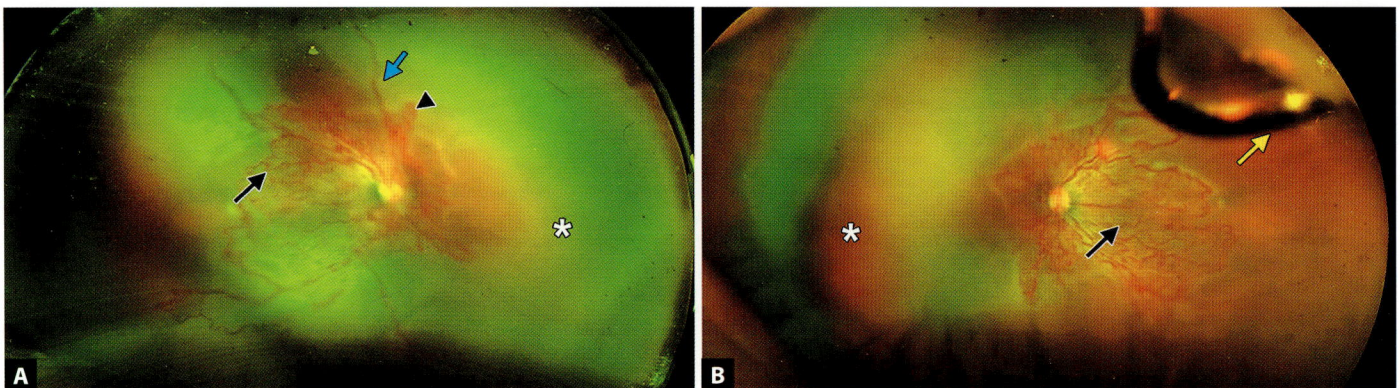

Figs. 1A and B: OU UWF fundus photos of baby with 32 weeks PMA, 28 weeks GA and 1.2 kg BW showing severe tortuosity of posterior pole vasculature (zone I) (black arrow), neovascular fronds (black short arrow), and looping of vessels (blue arrow) and ill-formed macula. The rest of the extensive area shows an avascular retina (asterisks). Both eyes received intravitreal bevacizumab injection. OS superior periphery shows a speculum artifact (yellow arrow). (BW: birth weight; GA: gestational age; OS: left eye; OU: both eyes; PMA: postmenstrual age; UWF: ultra-wide field)

■ BOTH EYES AGGRESSIVE RETINOPATHY OF PREMATURITY (Scenario 2)

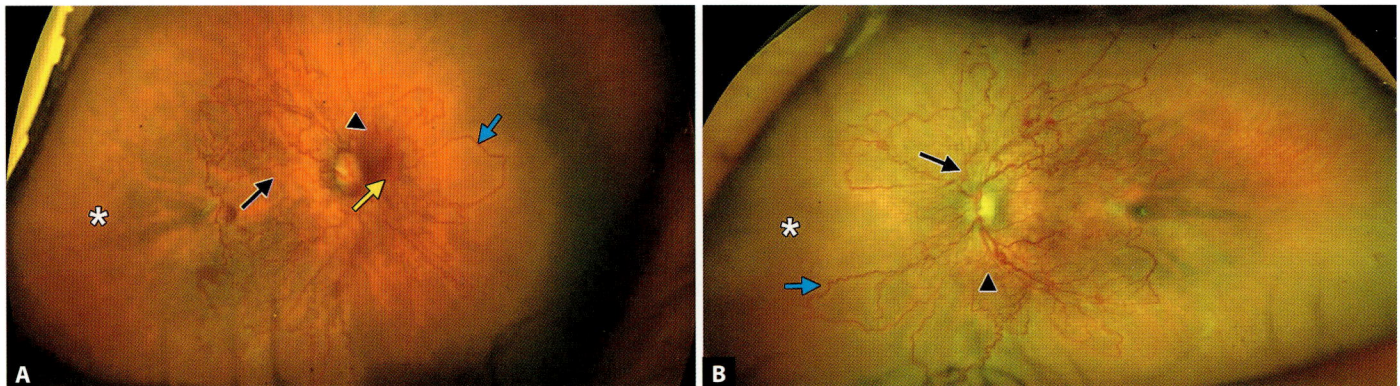

Figs. 2A and B: OU UWF fundus photos of baby with 36 weeks PMA, 32 weeks of GA and 1.6 kg BW showing severe tortuosity of posterior pole vasculature (zone I, 2p) (black arrow), neovascular fronds (black short arrow), preretinal hemorrhage in OD (yellow arrow) and looping of vessels (blue arrow). Rest of area shows is avascular retina (asterisks). Both eyes received panretinal laser photocoagulation. (BW: birth weight; GA: gestational age; OD: right eye; OU: both eyes; PMA: postmenstrual age; UWF: ultra-wide field)

STAGED RETINOPATHY OF PREMATURITY: ZONES, STAGES, AND TYPES

The recent International Classification of Retinopathy of Prematurity, Third Edition (ICROP3) guidelines describe retinal vascularization through three concentric circles of retinal zones extending till the ora serrata with optic disc as the center. Zone I is denoted by a circle with a radius twice the estimated distance from the optic disc center to the foveal center.

Zone II is the ring-shaped region extending nasally from the outer limit of zone I to the nasal ora serrata and with a similar distance temporally, superiorly, and inferiorly. Further zone II can be described as posterior zone II which is a region of two disc diameters peripheral to the zone I border. The newly introduced term "notch" will be subsequently discussed. Zone III is the residual crescent of the peripheral retina that extends beyond zone II where the nasal vessels are vascularized to the ora serrata and ROP is not present in the 2 nasal-most clock hours.

International Classification of Retinopathy of Prematurity, Third Edition has described stage 1 as the presence of a demarcation line, stage 2 with formation ridge, and stage 3 with the presence of extraretinal neovascular proliferation or flat neovascularization.

Stage 4: 4A with partial retinal detachment without involving the fovea, 4B with a detached fovea. Stage 5.5A, with open funnel total retinal detachment (optic disc is visible), 5B with closed-funnel detachment; and stage 5C, is with anterior segment changes such as marked anterior chamber shallowing, iridocorneolenticular adhesions, and corneal opacification along with changes of 5B.

Depending on the need of active intervention, staged ROP is divided into type 1, which involves eyes requiring active treatment, and type 2 in which close observation is recommended.[4]

■ RETINAL ZONES

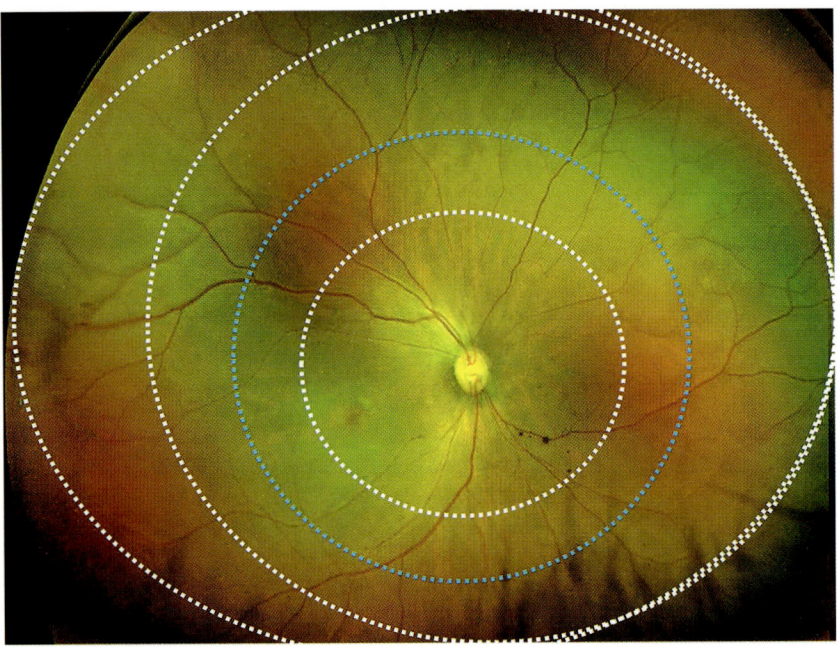

Fig. 3: OD UWF color fundus photo of pictorially depicting all four zones. Zone I extends till inner most white circle. Zone II posterior (recent addition by ICROP3) extends till blue circle. Zone II anterior extends till the middle white circle and zone III extends till the outermost white circle. (OD: right eye; UWF: ultra-wide field)

PLUS AND PREPLUS DISEASE

Retinal vascular changes in ROP occurs in a continuous spectrum from normal to preplus to plus disease. ICROP3 has defined Plus disease by the appearance of dilation and tortuosity of retinal vessels, where changes are assessed by the vessel changes within zone I and not merely based on vessels within the field of narrow-angle photographs or from the number of quadrants of abnormality. Preplus disease is defined by abnormal vascular dilation, tortuosity insufficient for plus disease, or both.

It is important to remember that the signs such as vascular engorgement of the iris, poor pupillary dilation, and peripheral retinal vascular engorgement with vitreous haze need not be always present in a plus disease; such signs are considered to occur in the advanced disease but are not necessary for the diagnosis of plus disease.[5]

LEFT EYE STAGE 1, ZONE II, PREPLUSE-TYPE 2

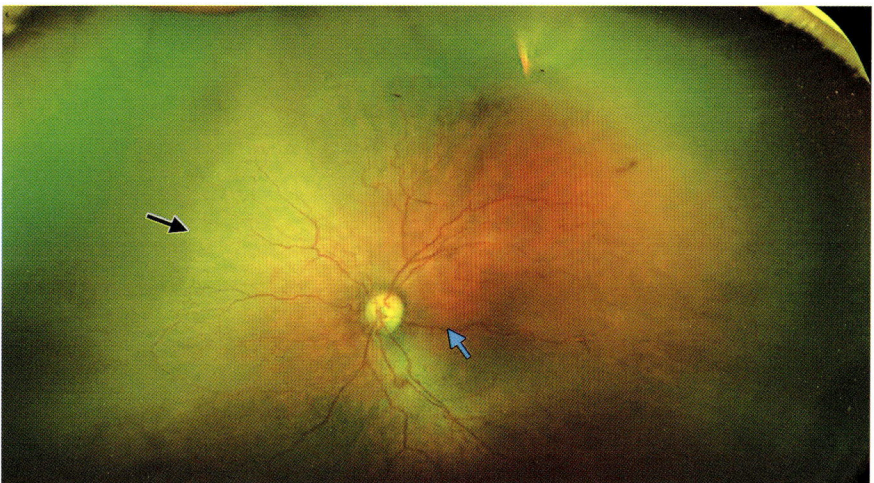

Fig. 4: OS UWF fundus photos of baby with 32 weeks PMA, 28 weeks of GA, and 1,000 g BW showing faint demarcation line (black arrow) in zone II posterior with mild tortuosity of vessels in posterior pole (blue arrow). A close follow-up is required in such eyes (type 2). (BW: birth weight; GA: gestational age; OS: left eye; PMA: postmenstrual age; UWF: ultra-wide field)

■ RIGHT EYE STAGE 3, ZONE II, LEFT EYE STAGE 2, ZONE II, BOTH EYES PREPLUS-TYPE 2

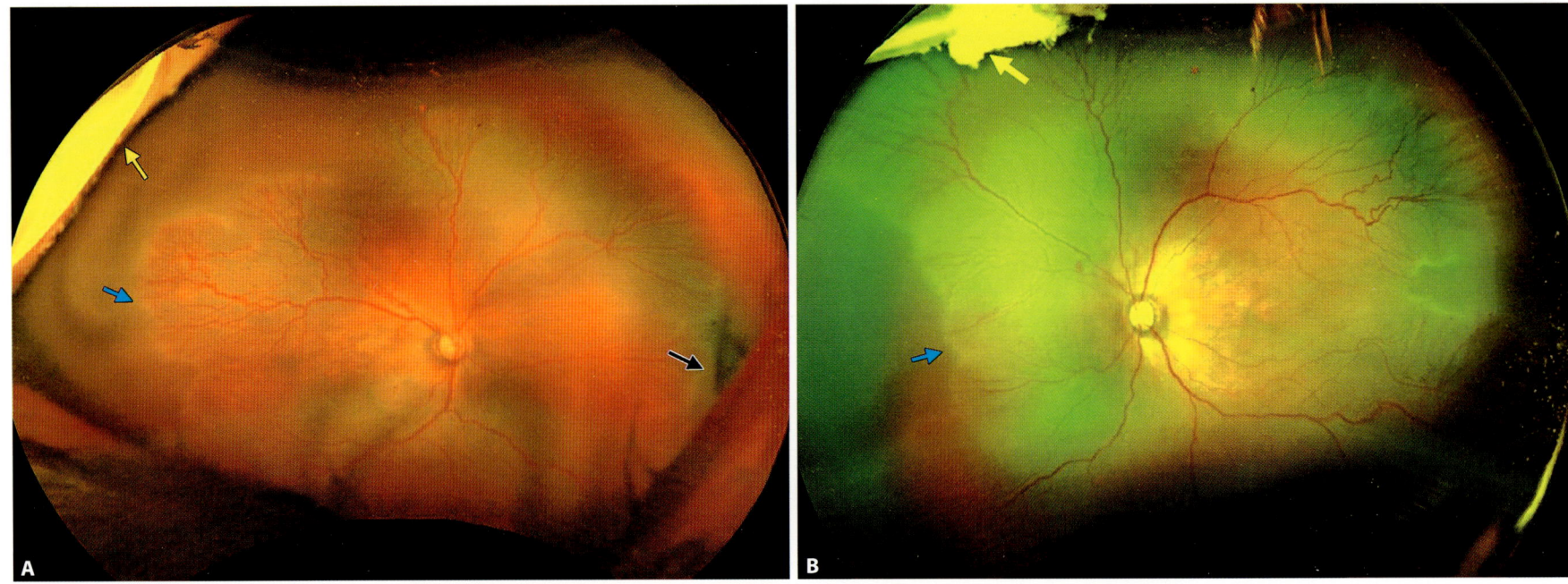

Figs. 5A and B: OU UWF fundus photos of baby with 33 weeks PMA, 26 weeks GA, and 1,200 g BW showing elevated ridge <2'O clock hour in nasal zone II anterior (black arrow) in OD and both the eyes having well demarcated ridge (blue arrow) and mildly tortuous posterior pole vessels. It is important to consider the finding which is in the posterior most zones and the presence of advanced stage when denoting the stages and zones. In this case OD posterior most zones has the advanced to stage III was in zone II. OU has aperture artifact (yellow arrow). Close follow-up is required in such cases to look for the progression (type 2). (BW: birth weight; GA: gestational age; OD: right eye; OU: both eyes; PMA: postmenstrual age; UWF: ultra-wide field)

BOTH EYES STAGE 2, ZONE II, AND PREPLUS-TYPE 2

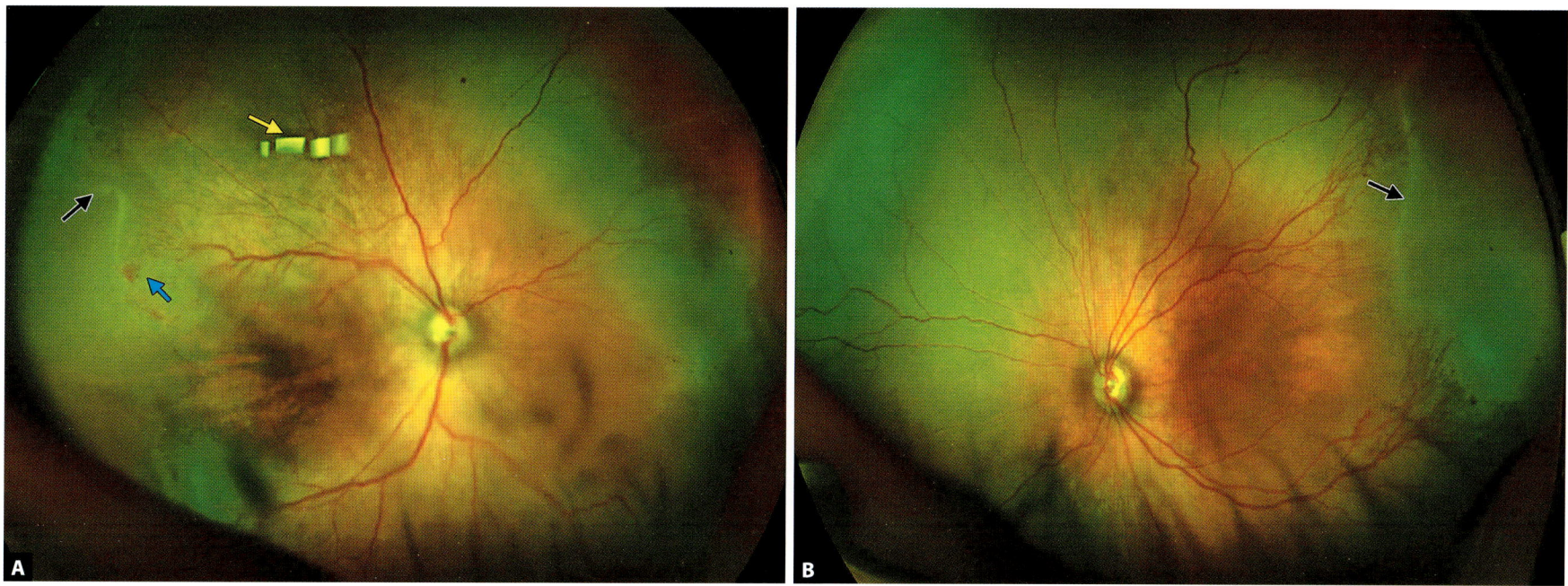

Figs. 6A and B: OU UWF fundus photos of baby with 34 weeks PMA, 29 weeks GA, and 1,170 g BW showing flat ridge in zone II posterior (black arrow) with mild tortuosity in posterior pole vessels. OD has flat hemorrhages (blue arrow) at the junction of the ridge and avascular retina. Such eye needs close follow-up (type 2). OD photo shows reflection artifact (yellow arrow). (BW: birth weight; GA: gestational age; OD: right eye; PMA: postmenstrual age; UWF: ultra-wide field)

■ BOTH EYES STAGE 2, ZONE II, WITH PLUS-TYPE 1

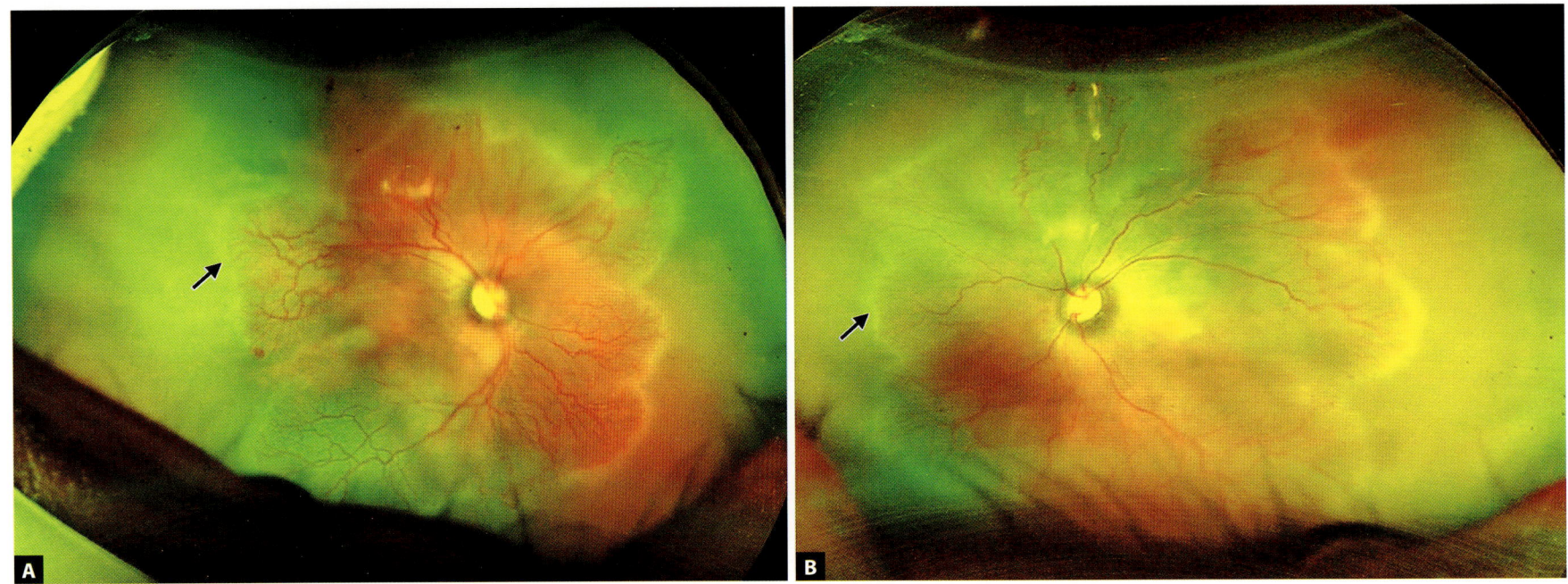

Figs. 7A and B: OU UWF fundus photos of baby with 32 weeks PMA, 28 weeks GA, and 1,100 g BW showing angry looking tortuous posterior and peripheral vessels (plus disease) with flat ridge in zone II posterior (black arrows). Note that media is clear with well dilated pupil. Such eyes needs early laser photocoagulation (type 1). (BW: birth weight; GA: gestational age; OU: both eyes; PMA: postmenstrual age; UWF: ultra-wide field)

■ RIGHT EYE STAGE 2, ZONE III ANTERIOR, PREPLUS-TYPE 2

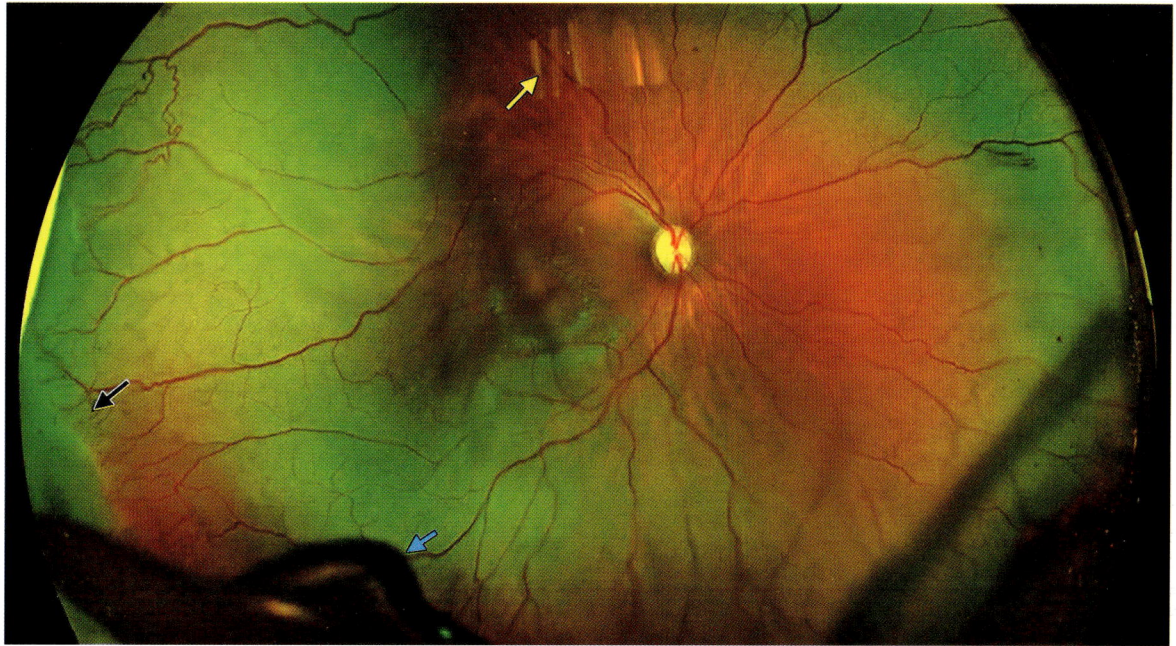

Fig. 8: OD UWF fundus photos of baby with 42 weeks PMA, 38 weeks GA, and 2,100 g BW showing flat ridge in zone III anterior (black arrow), with completely vascularized zone II. Note the vessels in periphery looks more tortuous but posterior pole vessel tortuosity is mild. Speculum artifact (blue arrow) and reflection artifact (yellow arrow) can be seen. (BW: birth weight; GA: gestational age; OD: right eye; PMA: postmenstrual age; UWF: ultra-wide field)

■ BOTH EYES, STAGE 2, ZONE II ANTERIOR, NO PLUS-TYPE 2

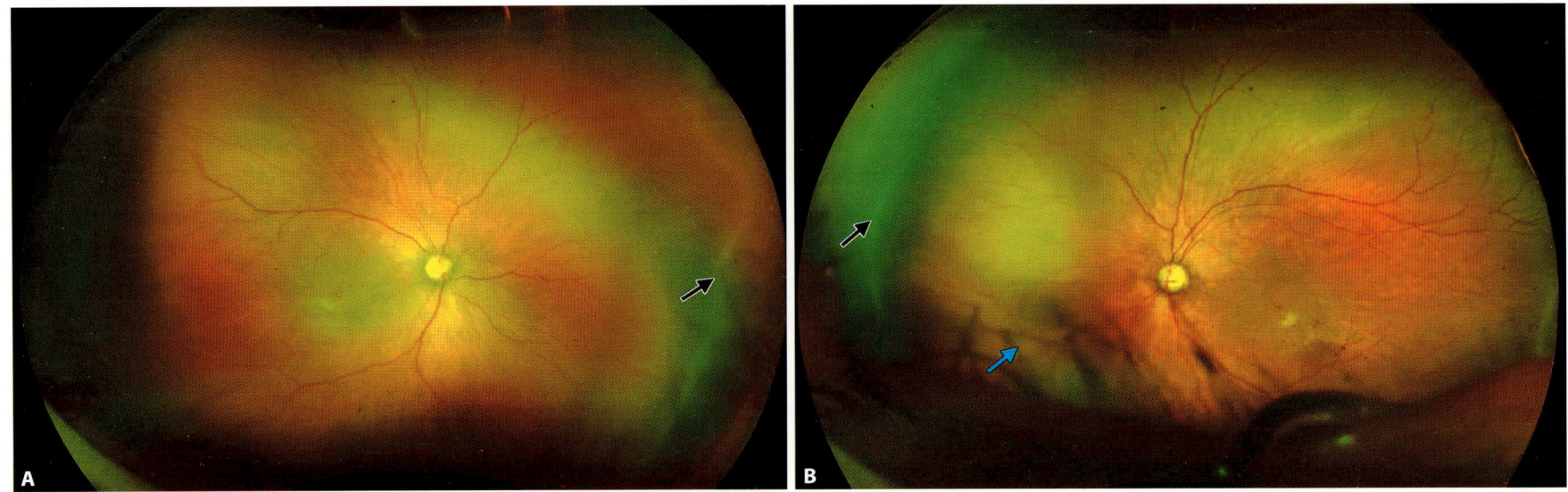

Figs. 9A and B: OU UWF fundus photos of baby with 37 weeks PMA, 29 weeks GA, and 840 g BW with flat ridge in zone II (black arrow) with normal posterior pole vessel couture. Eye lash artifact (blue arrow) can be seen. (BW: birth weight; GA: gestational age; OU: both eyes; PMA: postmenstrual age; UWF: ultra-wide field)

■ RIGHT EYE STAGE 2, LEFT EYE, STAGE 3 IN ZONE II WITH PLUS-TYPE 1

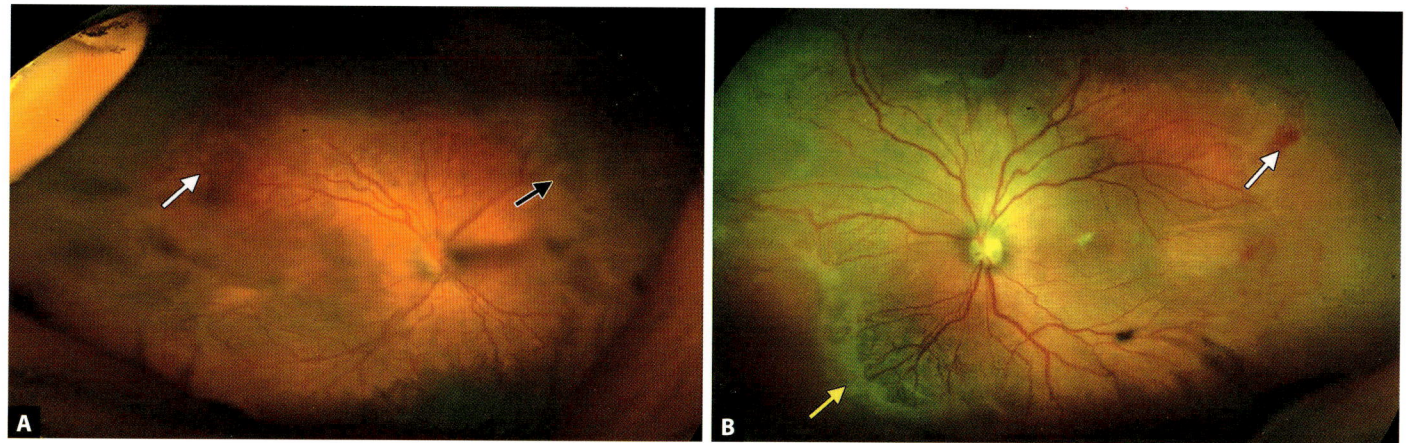

Figs. 10A and B: OU UWF fundus photos of baby with 36 weeks PMA, 33 weeks GA, and 809 g BW showing OD faint ridge in zone II posterior (black arrow), OS elevated ridge 2–3'O clock hour in inferonasal quadrant of zone II (yellow arrow). OU have tortuous vessels in posterior pole and beyond with few flat hemorrhages (white arrow). (BW: birth weight; GA: gestational age; OD: right eye; OS: left eye; OU: both eyes; PMA: postmenstrual age; UWF: ultra-wide field)

■ BOTH EYES STAGE 3, ZONE II, AND PLUS-TYPE 1

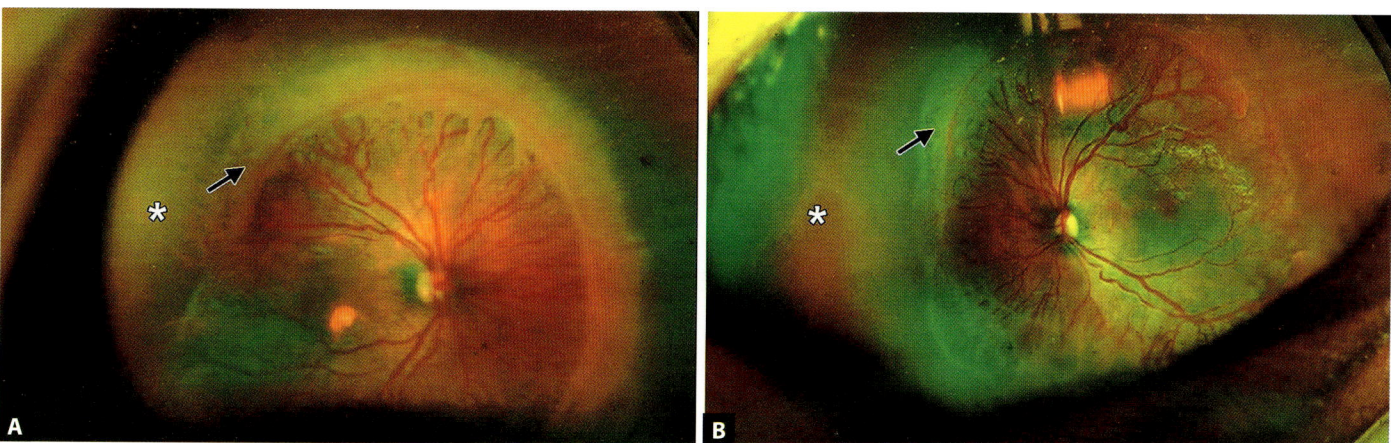

Figs. 11A and B: OU UWF fundus photos of baby with 34 weeks PMA, 29 weeks GA, and 1,280 g BW showing elevated ridge across zone II (black arrow) with severe dilatation and tortuosity of entire retinal vessels. A total avascular retina can be seen beyond the ridge (asterisks). (BW: birth weight; GA: gestational age; OU: both eye; OU: both eyes; PMA: postmenstrual age; UWF: ultra-wide field)

BOTH EYES STAGE 3, ZONE II WITH RIGHT EYE PRERETINAL HEMORRHAGE, AND LEFT EYE ELEVATED RIDGE WITH UNDERLYING FLAT RETINA-TYPE 1

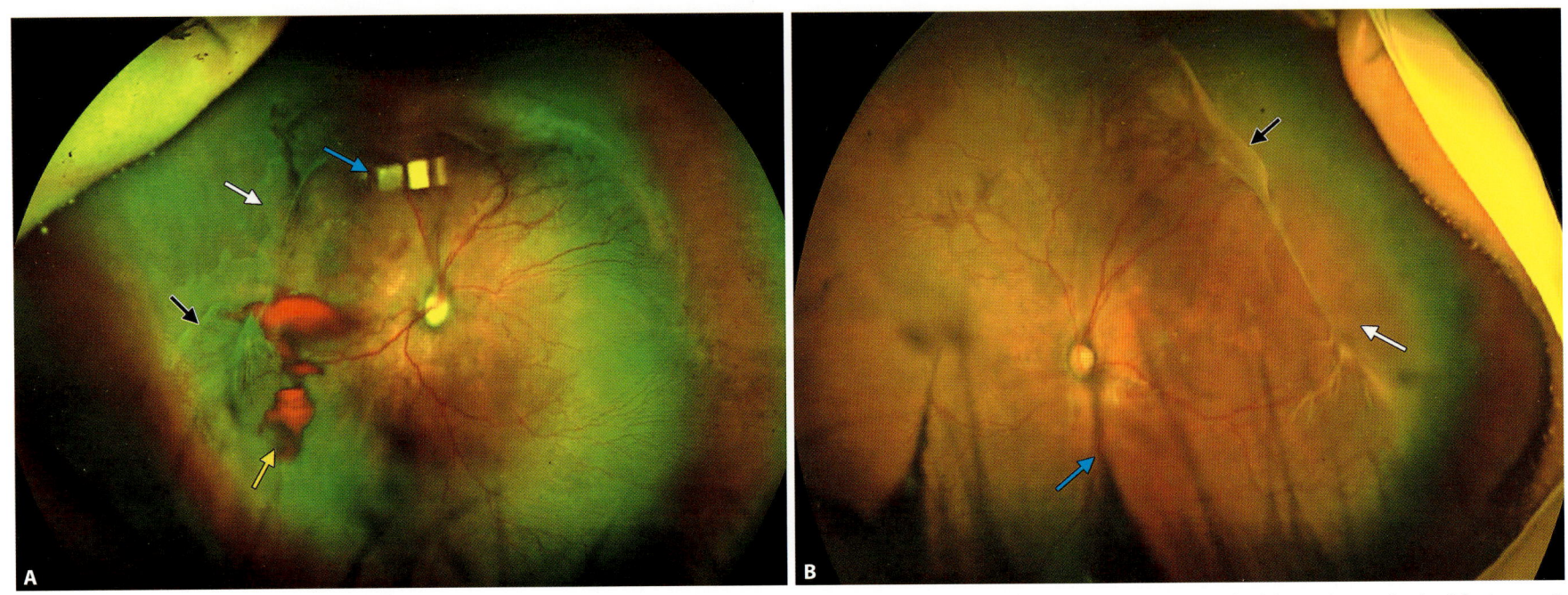

Figs. 12A and B: OU UWF fundus photos of baby with 37 weeks PMA, 28 weeks GA, and 900 g BW, showing elevated ridge in zone II >3 'O clock hours in continuity (black arrow). A preretinal hemorrhage along the ridge can be seen in OD (yellow arrow). OS shows extending flat retina beyond the ridge margins (white arrow). Reflection and eyelash artifacts can be seen (blue arrow). (BW: birth weight; GA: gestational age; OD: right eye; OS: left eye; OU: both eyes; PMA: postmenstrual age; UWF: ultra-wide field)

■ RIGHT EYE STAGE 4B, LEFT EYE STAGE 4A WITH PRERETINAL HEMORRHAGE BOTH EYES

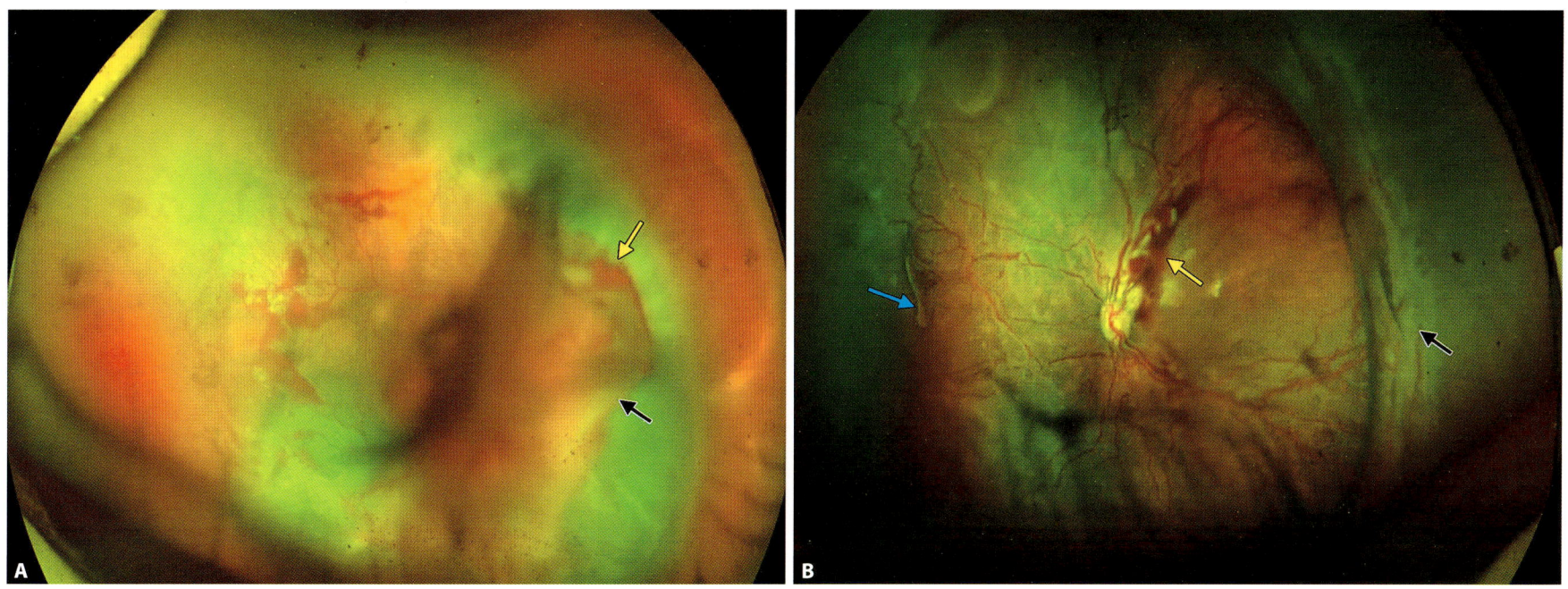

Figs. 13A and B: OU UWF fundus photos of baby with 39 weeks PMA, 28 weeks GA, and 960 g BW showing OD tractional retinal detachment involving fovea (black arrow) with vitreous hemorrhage (yellow arrow). OS has also tractional detachment (black arrow) temporally without involving fovea and a flat ridge in nasal quadrant (blue arrow). Preretinal hemorrhage near disc can be seen (yellow arrow). (BW: birth weight; GA: gestational age; OD: right eye; OS: left eye; OU: both eyes; PMA: postmenstrual age; UWF: ultra-wide field)

STAGE 4A WITH PRERETINAL HEMORRHAGE

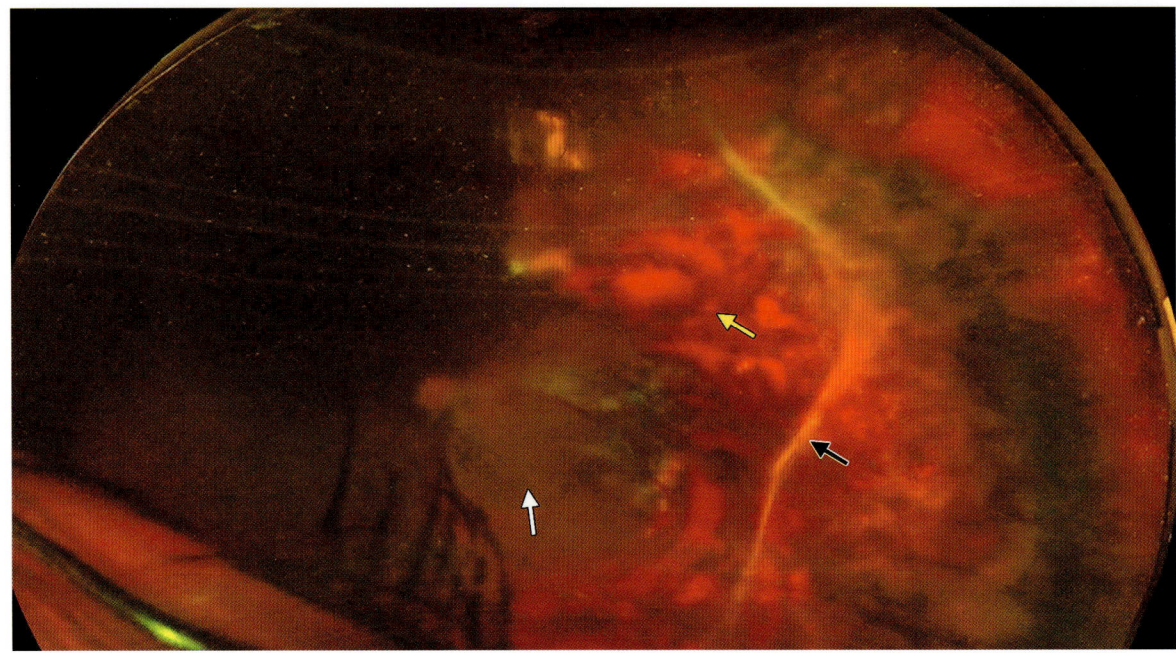

Fig. 14: OD UWF fundus photos of baby with 36 weeks PMA, 28 weeks GA, and 1,160 g BW showing elevated ridge (black arrow) with extensive preretinal hemorrhage (yellow arrow) and an intact fovea (white arrow). (BW: birth weight; GA: gestational age; OD: right eye; PMA: postmenstrual age; UWF: ultra-wide field)

■ BOTH EYES STAGE 4B RETINOPATHY OF PREMATURITY

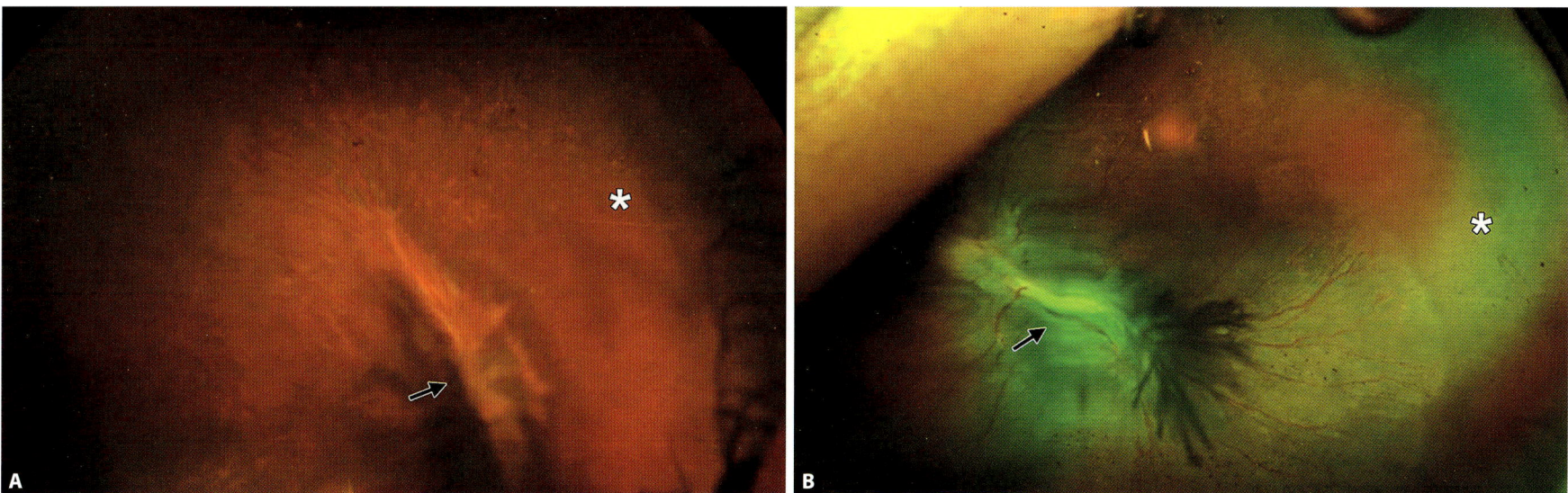

Figs. 15A and B: OU UWF fundus photos of baby with 40 weeks PMA, 28 weeks GA, and 1,200 g BW showing tractional detachment involving fovea (black arrow) along with extensive avascular retina in periphery (asterisks). (BW: birth weight; GA: gestational age; OU: both eyes; PMA: postmenstrual age; UWF: ultra-wide field)

■ REFERENCES

1. Chiang MF, Quinn GE, Fielder AR, Ostmo SR, Paul Chan RV, Berrocal A, et al. International Classification of Retinopathy of Prematurity, Third Edition. Ophthalmology. 2021;128(10):e51-68.
2. International Committee for the Classification of Retinopathy of Prematurity. The International Classification of Retinopathy of Prematurity revisited. Arch Ophthalmol. 2005;123(7):991-9.
3. Sanghi G, Dogra MR, Katoch D, Gupta A. Aggressive posterior retinopathy of prematurity in infants ≥1500 g birth weight. Indian J Ophthalmol. 2014;62(2):254-7.
4. Early Treatment For Retinopathy Of Prematurity Cooperative Group. Revised indications for the treatment of retinopathy of prematurity: results of the early treatment for retinopathy of prematurity randomized trial. Arch Ophthalmology. 2003;121(12):1684-94.
5. An international classification of retinopathy of prematurity. The Committee for the Classification of Retinopathy of Prematurity. Arch Ophthalmol. 1984;102(8):1130-4.

CHAPTER 3

Peculiar Findings in Retinopathy of Prematurity

■ INTRODUCTION

Amidst the common clinical presentations of ROP, certain peculiar signs can offer unique insights into the pathophysiology, prognosis, and management. This chapter throws light on few such distinctive findings and their significance.

■ "POPCORN" AND "HOT DOG"-LIKE HEMORRHAGES

"Popcorn"-like hemorrhages are small isolated yellowish white round tufts of neovascular tissue on the surface of the retina usually seen posterior to the stage II ridge in zone II. Presence of these lesion is one of the features of regression of the disease;[1] however, spontaneous regression of retinopathy of prematurity (ROP) with popcorn lesions is longer than those without these lesions.[2]

"Hot dog"-like linear red lesions over the thickened vascular ridge with no typical fronds of neovascularization, seen over the stage II ridge in zone II. It is one of the signs for disease progression and a poor prognostic indicator.[3]

■ "RIDGE DOUBLING" AND "NOTCH SIGN"

Ridge doubling is seen in staged ROP where two ridges can be made out usually in zone II, one anterior which is moving toward zone III, and the other posterior which can be either elevated or regressing with avulsed vessels floating in the vitreous. The presence of ridge doubling is a sign of progression of the disease.[4] Notch sign is recently added in the International Classification of Retinopathy of Prematurity, Third Edition (ICROP3) by the classification committee, describing it as an incursion by the ROP lesion of 1–2 clock hours along the horizontal meridian into a more posterior zone than the remainder of the retinopathy. It has to be recorded as the most posterior zone of retinal vascularization with the qualifier "secondary to notch."[5]

RIGHT EYE POPCORN-LIKE LESIONS WITH STAGE 2 ZONE II, PREPLUS-TYPE 2

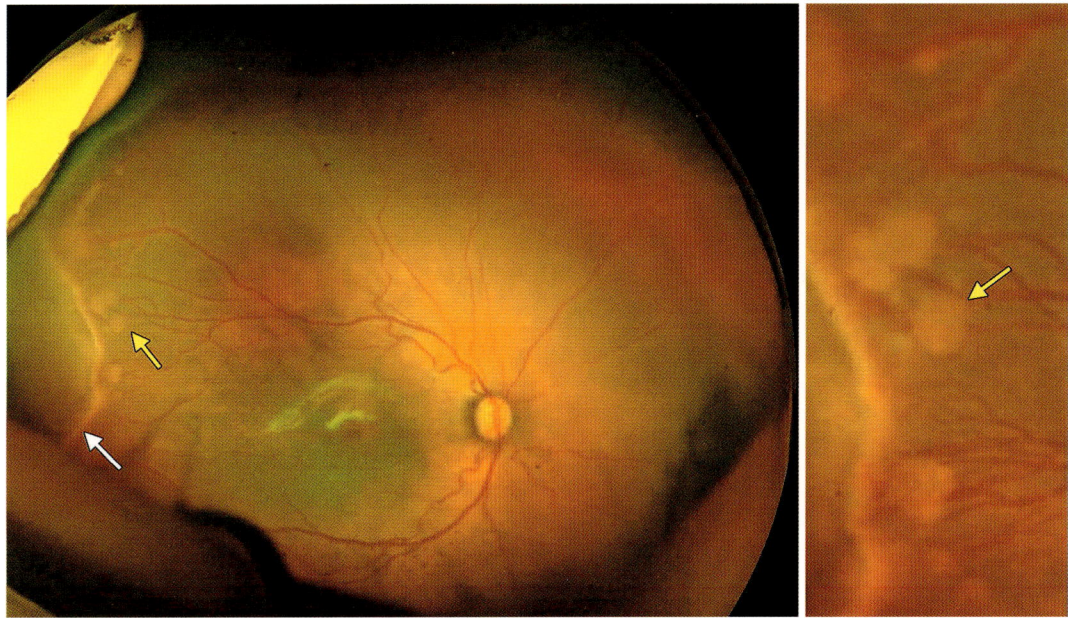

Fig. 1: UWF fundus photos of OD 34 weeks PMA baby with 29 weeks GA and 1,200 g BW showing small round whitish popcorn-like old hemorrhages (yellow arrow) along the flat ridge (white arrow). Inset—magnified image of the temporal lesions. (BW: birth weight; GA: gestational age; OD: right eye; PMA: postmenstrual age; UWF: ultra-wide field)

LEFT EYE HOT DOG-LIKE LINEAR HEMORRHAGE ALONG THE RIDGE, STAGE 3, ZONE II, PREPLUS-TYPE 2

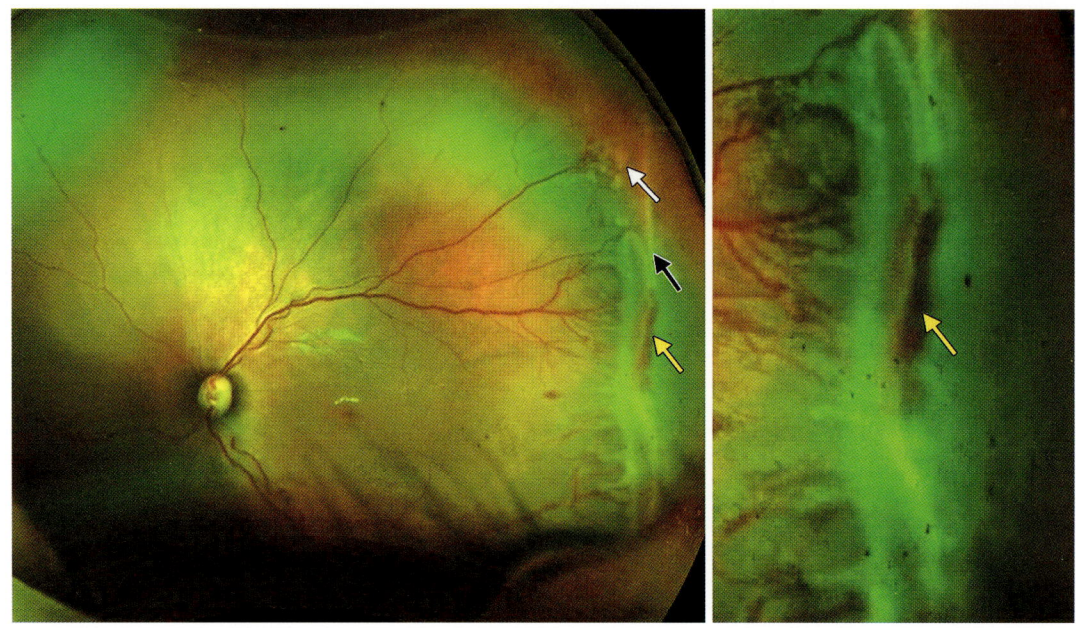

Fig. 2: UWF fundus photos of OS 36 weeks PMA baby with 29 weeks GA, and 1,200 g BW showing elevated ridge (black arrow) with linear hemorrhages over the ridge appearing like a "hotdog" (yellow arrow) along with some popcorn hemorrhages (white arrow). Inset: Magnified view of temporal linear hemorrhage. (BW: birth weight; GA: gestational age; OS: left eye; PMA: postmenstrual age; UWF: ultra-wide field)

RIGHT EYE RIDGE DOUBLING, STAGE 3, ZONE II, PLUS-TYPE 1

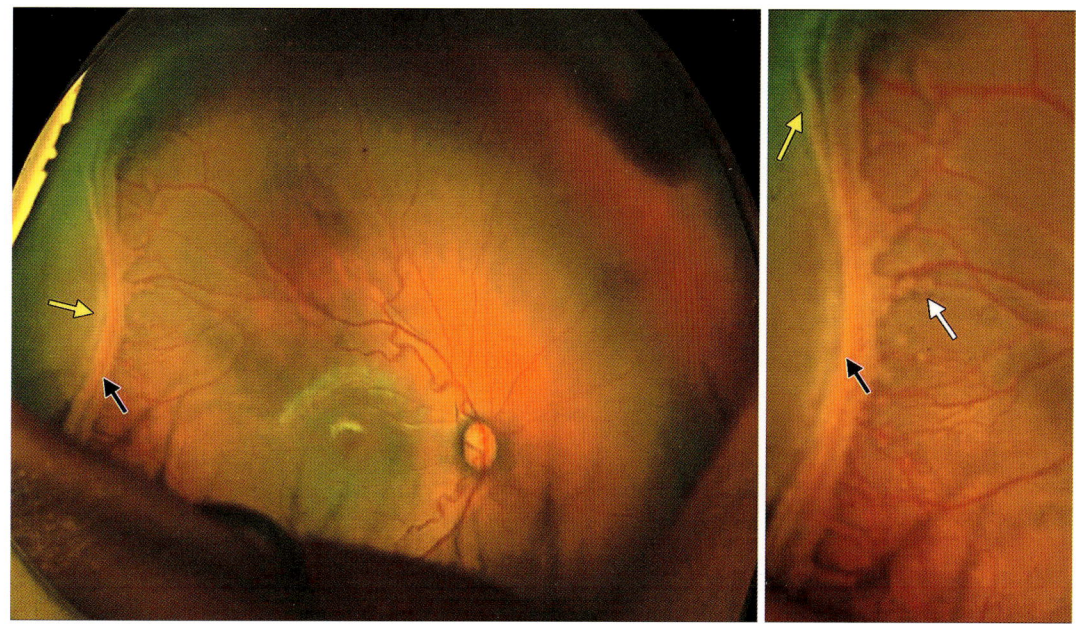

Fig. 3: UWF fundus photos of OD 36 weeks PMA baby with 29 weeks GA and 1,200 g BW showing elevated ridge <3 contiguous clock hour posterior (black arrow) and a flat ridge anterior to it (yellow arrow) forming a pattern of "ridge doubling." Dilated and tortuous retinal vessels in posterior pole and beyond can be seen. Inset—temporal image is the magnified view showing doubling of ridge along with popcorn lesions (white arrows). (BW: birth weight; GA: gestational age; OD: right eye; PMA: postmenstrual age; UWF: ultra-wide field)

RIGHT EYE RIDGE DOUBLING, REGRESSING FROM STAGE 3 TO STAGE 2, ZONE III-TYPE 2 (POSTERIOR RIDGE AND ANTERIOR FLAT RETINA)

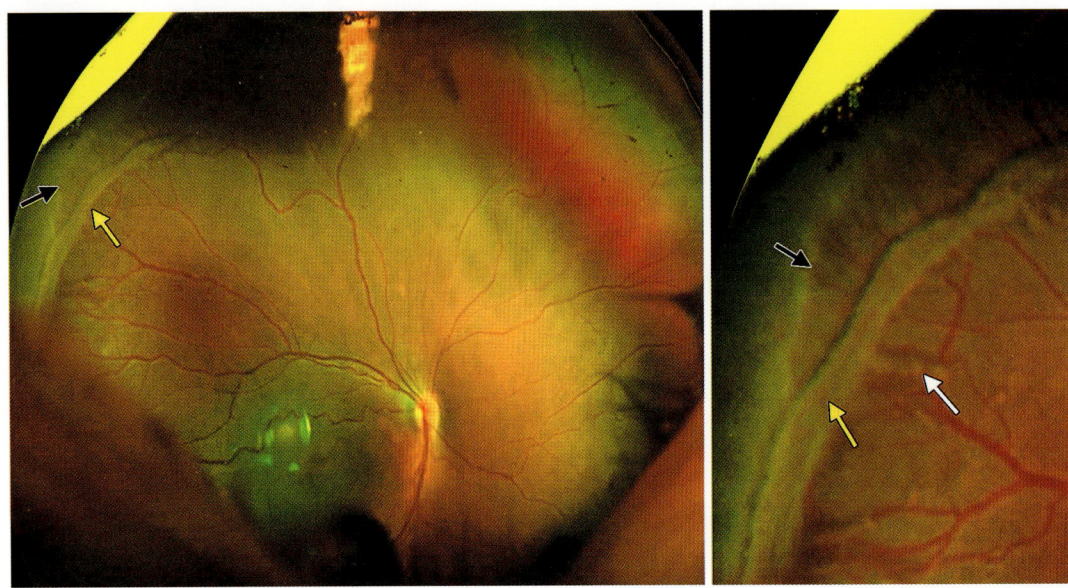

Fig. 4: UWF fundus photos of OD 34 weeks PMA baby with 27 weeks GA and 990 g BW showing ridge doubling with flat anterior ridge (black arrow) with regressing posterior ridge elevation (yellow arrow) and mild tortuosity of vessels. Inset—magnified view of doubling of the ridge with few popcorn lesions (white arrow). (BW: birth weight; GA: gestational age; OD: right eye; PMA: postmenstrual age; UWF: ultra-wide field)

■ LEFT EYE RIDGE DOUBLING WITH POPCORNS IN STAGE 2, ZONE II, PREPLUS-TYPE 2

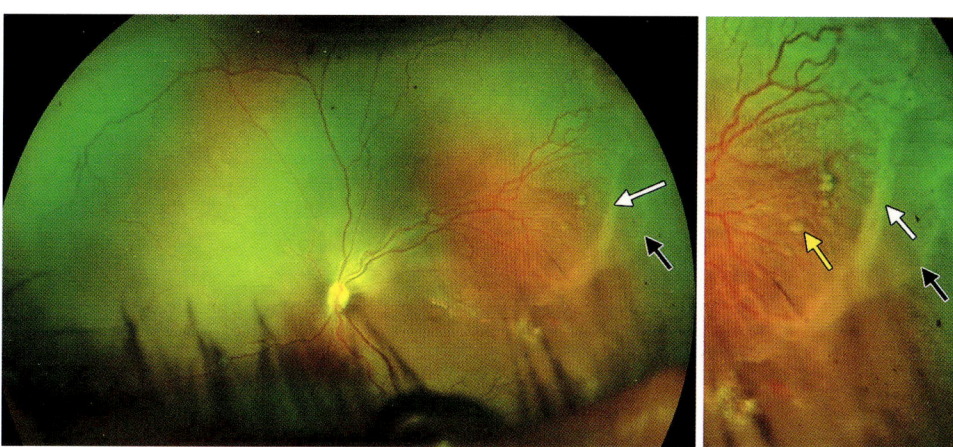

Fig. 5: UWF fundus photos of OS 33 weeks PMA baby with 28 weeks GA and 1,000 g BW with ridge doubling showing both anterior (black arrow) and posterior flat ridge (white arrow) in zone II and mild tortuosity of vessels. Inset—magnified view of the ridge doubling with popcorn lesions (yellow arrow). (BW: birth weight; GA: gestational age; OS: left eye; PMA: postmenstrual age; UWF: ultra-wide field)

■ LEFT EYE AVULSED VESSELS WITH REGRESSING RIDGE AND FLAT RETINA ANTERIOR TO RIDGE, STAGE 3, ZONE II, PREPLUS-TYPE 2

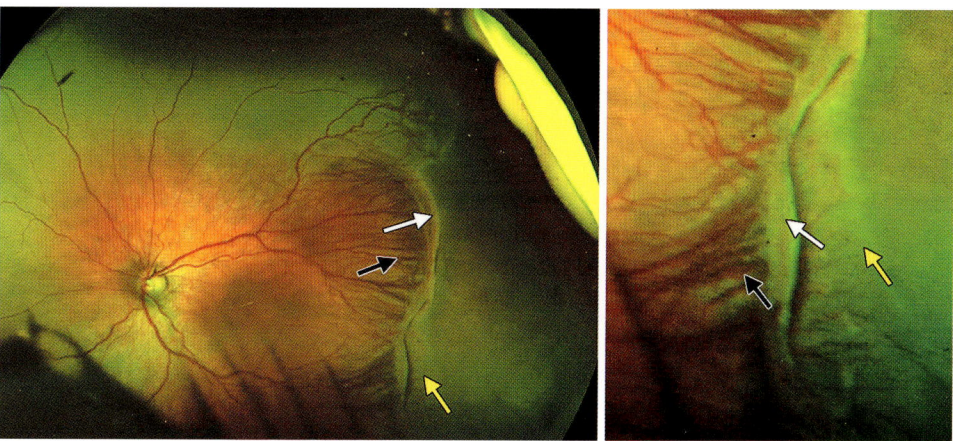

Fig. 6: UWF fundus photos of OS 34 weeks PMA baby with 29 weeks GA, and 1,200 g BW showing the avulsed floating vessels (black arrow) along the regressing posterior elevated ridge (white arrow) and flat anterior ridge (yellow arrow). Inset: Magnified temporal image to show avulsed vessels along with ridge doubling. (BW: birth weight; GA: gestational age; OS: left eye; PMA: postmenstrual age; UWF: ultra-wide field)

RIGHT EYE RIDGE NOTCHING, STAGE 2, ZONE II, NO PLUS-TYPE 2

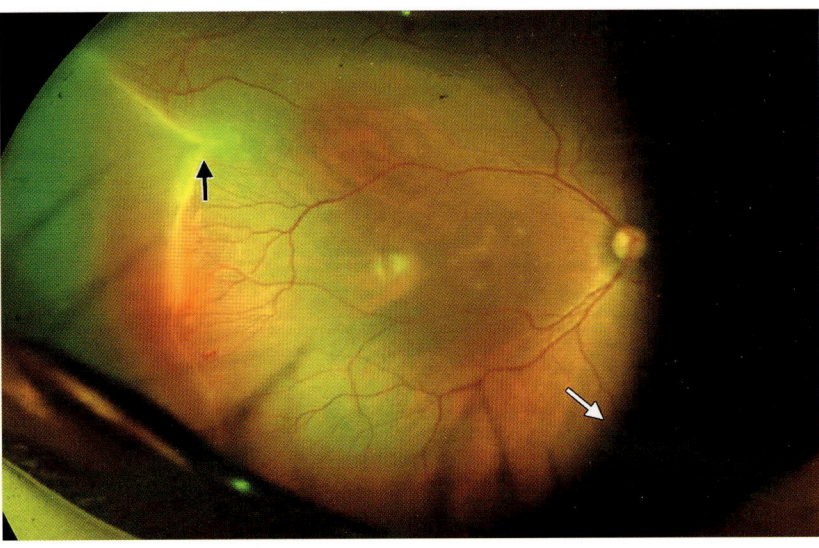

Fig. 7: UWF fundus photos of OD 38 weeks PMA baby with 30 weeks GA and 1,100 g BW showing notch extending to zone II (black arrow) described as "zone II secondary to notch." A shadow artefact from the aperture can be seen nasally (white arrow). (BW: birth weight; GA: gestational age; OD: right eye; PMA: postmenstrual age; UWF: ultra-wide field)

■ LEFT EYE RIDGE NOTCHING IN POSTERIOR POLE, STAGE 2, ZONE II PLUS-TYPE 1

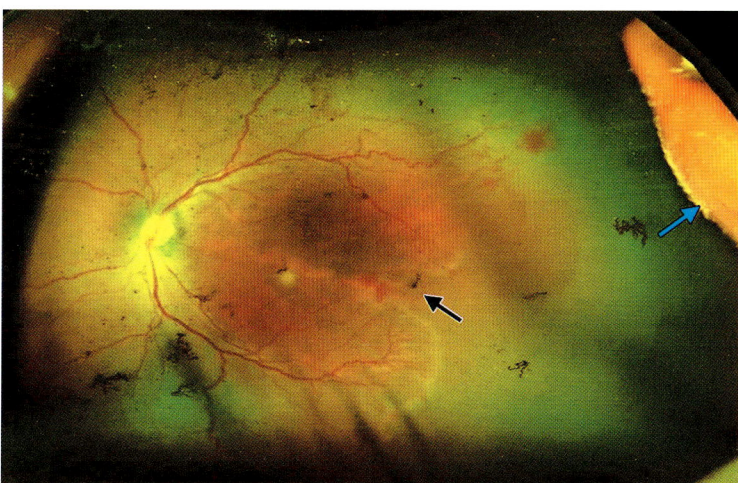

Fig. 8: UWF fundus photos of OS 32 weeks PMA baby with 28 weeks GA, and 1,000 g BW showing the notch sign extending to zone I (black arrow) described as "zone I secondary to notch" with tortuous vessels. A nose artifact is seen in superotemporal quadrant (blue arrow). (BW: birth weight; GA: gestational age; OS: left eye; PMA: postmenstrual age; UWF: ultra-wide field)

■ LEFT EYE RIDGE NOTCHING IN POSTERIOR POLE, STAGE 2, ZONE II, PREPLUS-TYPE 2

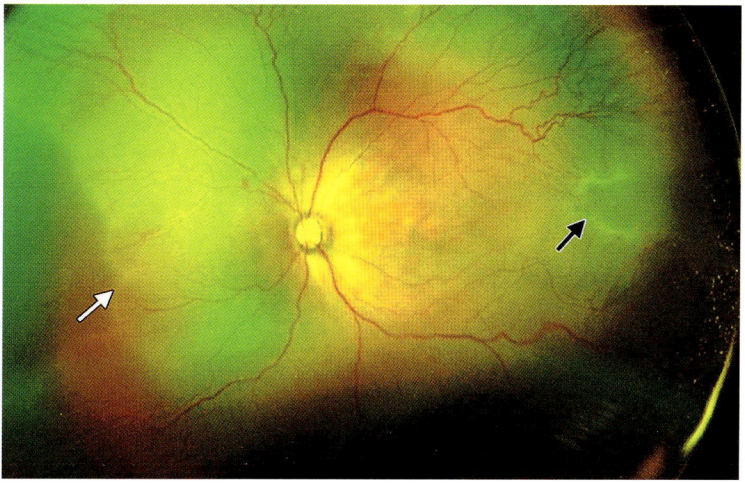

Fig. 9: UWF fundus photos of OS 33 weeks PMA baby with 26 weeks GA and 1,200 g BW with ridge in zone II (white arrow) with a temporal notch (black arrow) with mild tortuosity of vessels. (BW: birth weight; GA: gestational age; OS: left eye; PMA: postmenstrual age; UWF: ultra-wide field)

LEFT EYE ZONE III IMMATURE WITH SPONTANEOUS RESOLUTION OF VITREOUS HEMORRHAGE SECONDARY TO BIRTH RELATED TRAUMA IN 4 WEEKS

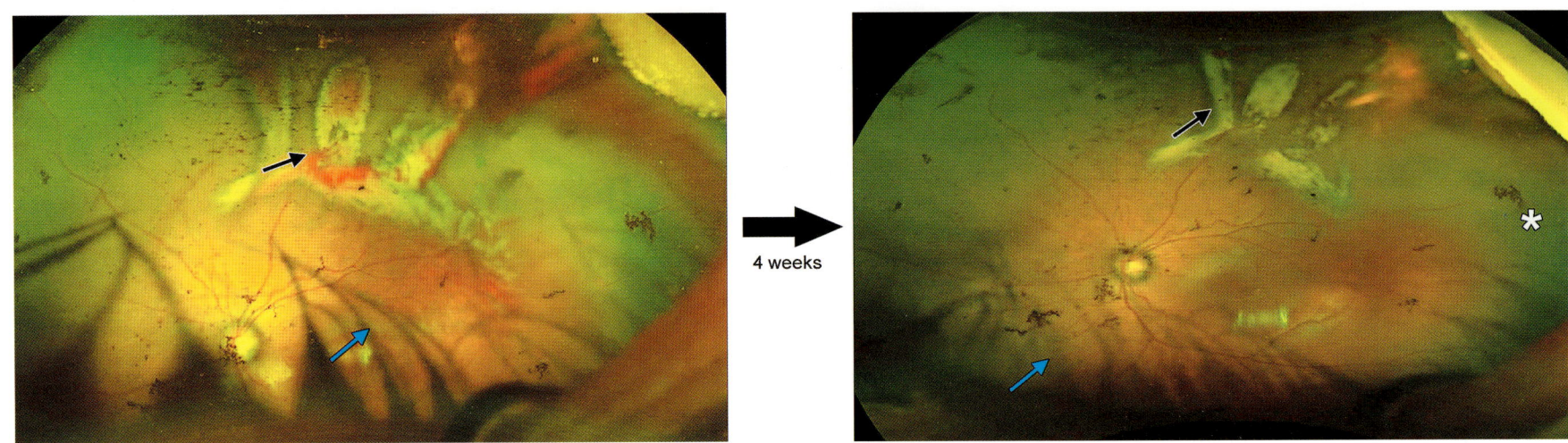

Fig. 10: UWF fundus photos of OS 38 weeks PMA baby with 30 weeks GA and 1,100 g BW with vitreous hemorrhage secondary to birth trauma (black arrow). It resolved spontaneously in 4 weeks (right mage) with immature retina in zone III (asterisks). Eye lash artefact is seen (blue arrow). (BW: birth weight; GA: gestational age; OS: left eye; PMA: postmenstrual age; UWF: ultra-wide field)

BOTH EYES PRERETINAL HEMORRHAGE DUE THROMBOCYTOPENIA

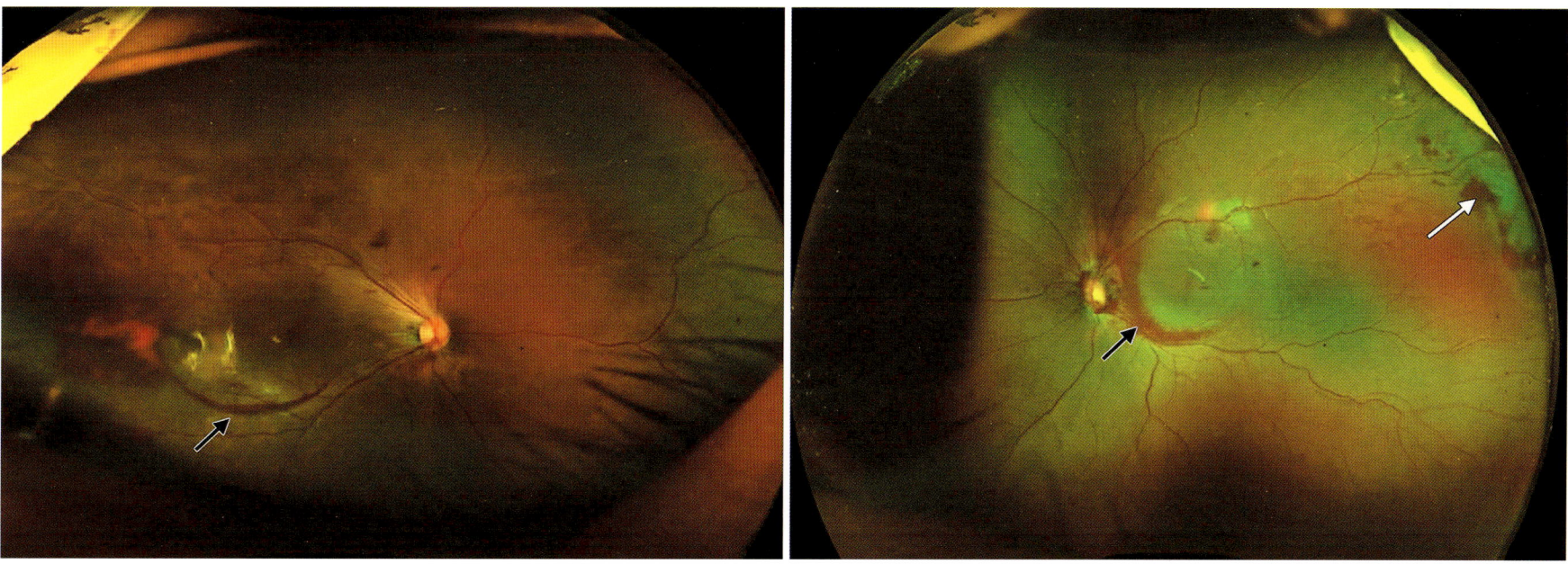

Fig. 11: UWF fundus photos of OU 40 weeks PMA baby with 32 weeks GA and 1,300 g BW with thrombocytopenia showing bilateral streaks preretinal hemorrhage in posterior pole (black arrow) and in periphery (white arrow) which is not related to ROP with near mature retina in zone III. (BW: birth weight; GA: gestational age; OU: both eyes; PMA: postmenstrual age; ROP: retinopathy of prematurity; UWF: ultra-wide field)

■ RIGHT EYE STAGE 2, ZONE II, PREPLUS WITH PRERETINAL BLEED AT THE FOVEA

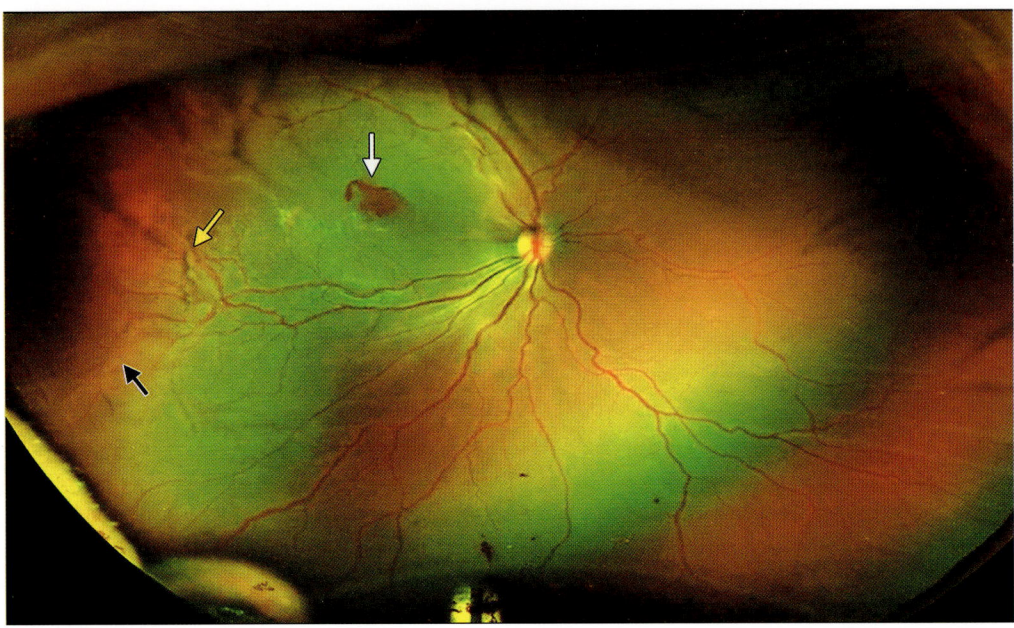

Fig. 12: UWF fundus photos of OD 36 weeks PMA baby with 28 weeks GA, and 1,200 g BW showing ridge in zone II (black arrow) with few popcorn hemorrhages (yellow arrow), mild tortuous retinal vessels, and a focal preretinal bleed at fovea (white arrow). (BW: birth weight; GA: gestational age; OD: right eye; PMA: postmenstrual age; ROP: retinopathy of prematurity; UWF: ultra-wide field)

BOTH EYES AGGRESSIVE RETINOPATHY OF PREMATURITY WITH EARLY FIBROVASCULAR PROLIFERATION AT DISC AND NASAL RETINA

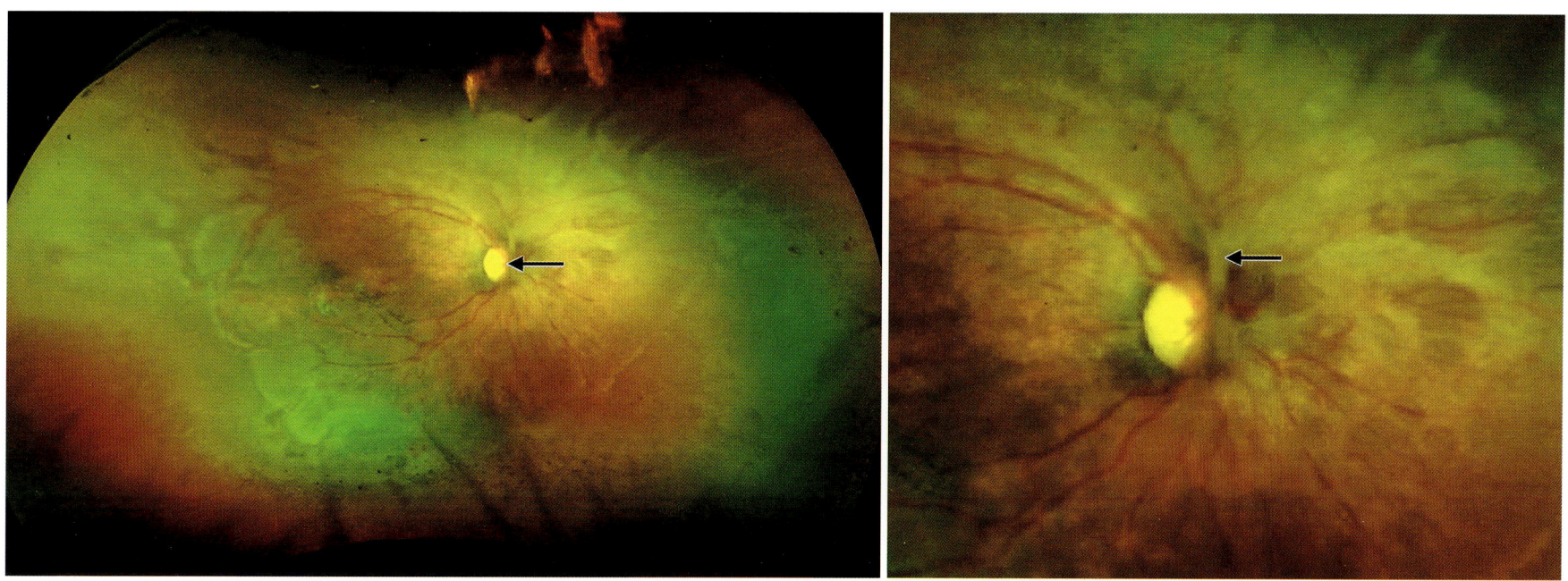

Fig. 13: UWF fundus photos of OD 38 weeks PMA baby with 32 weeks GA and 1,600 g BW with aggressive ROP with flat fibrous membranes in zone I. On a closer look (left image) membrane is seen extending from the disc (black arrow). Right image—magnified view of the peripapillary area. (BW: birth weight; GA: gestational age; OD: right eye; PMA: postmenstrual age; ROP: retinopathy of prematurity; UWF: ultra-wide field)

REFERENCES

1. Xue K, Huang X, Xu S, Zhang T, Wang X, Zhang M, et al. The evolution of isolated neovascular tufts ("popcorn") in retinopathy of prematurity. Retina. 2020;40(7):1353-8.
2. Wang L, Li M, Zhu J, Yan H, Wu L, Fan J, et al. Clinical Features of Spontaneous Regression of Retinopathy of Prematurity in China: A 5-Year Retrospective Case Series. Front Med (Lausanne). 2021;8:731421.
3. Kretzer FL, Hittner HM. Retinopathy of prematurity: clinical implications of retinal development. Arch Dis Child. 1988;63(10 Spec No):1151-67.
4. Yaz Y, Erol N, Gursoy H, Basmak H, Bilgec MD. A rare association of intravitreal bevacizumab injection with double ridge formation in retinopathy of prematurity. J Pediatric Ophthalmology Strabismus. 2014;51 Online:e66-8.
5. Chiang MF, Quinn GE, Fielder AR, Ostmo SR, Paul Chan RV, Berrocal A, et al. International Classification of Retinopathy of Prematurity, Third Edition. Ophthalmology. 2021;128(10):e51-68.

CHAPTER 4

Atypical Presentations of Retinopathy of Prematurity

■ INTRODUCTION

As clinicians, we are accustomed to visualize retinopathy of prematurity (ROP) as either aggressive retinopathy of prematurity (A-ROP) or staged ROP. Yet few uncommon presentations need to be familiarizes as it can alter the management and prognosis. This chapter helps in understanding such atypical presentations which can be a diagnostic challenge.

■ HALF ZONE RETINOPATHY OF PREMATURITY

Zone I, is defined as the posterior most region, and denoted by a circle with radius twice the estimated distance from the optic disc center to the foveal center. A-ROP usually involves tortuosity and new vessels in this zone and beyond.[1] In a few extremely premature babies, the vessels involved in A-ROP are less than the area of zone I description. These babies would have very poorly formed macula and fovea; this is termed as half zone ROP. These eyes usually require combined treatment [intravitreal antivascular endothelial growth factor (anti-VEGF) and laser photocoagulation].[1,2]

■ BOTH EYES HALF ZONE RETINOPATHY OF PREMATURITY

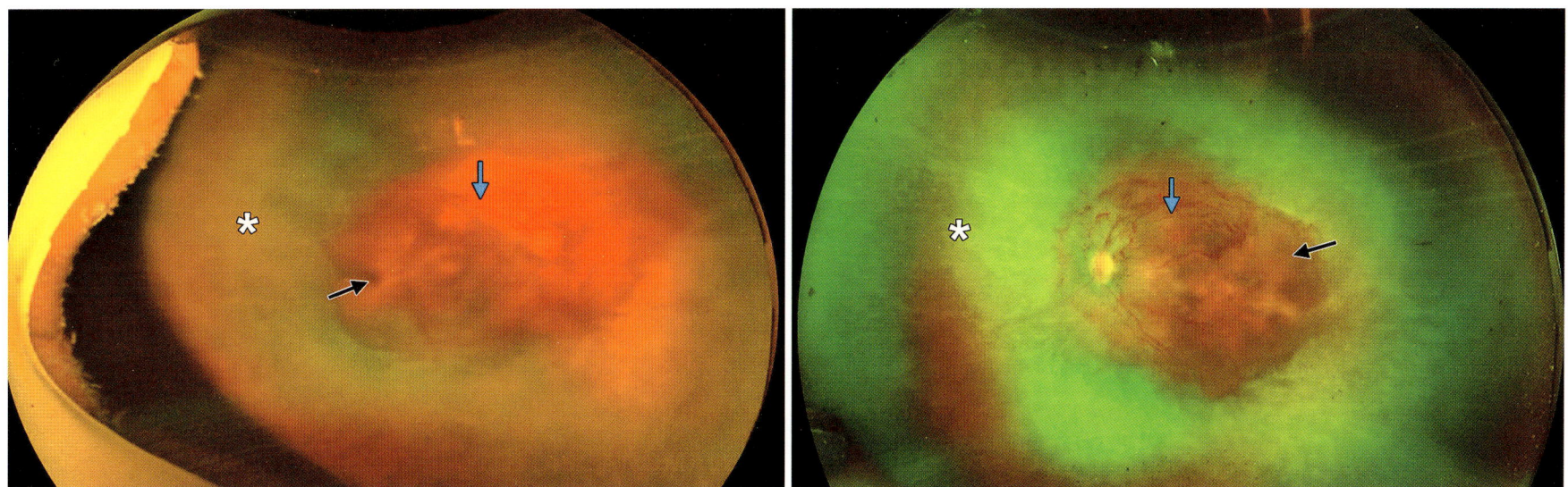

Fig. 1: UWF fundus photos of OU and of 34 weeks PMA baby with 28 weeks GA and 1,200 g BW showing vitreous hemorrhage (black arrow) with poorly formed macula and poorly formed arcade vessels with severe tortuosity (blue arrow). Rest of retina is completely avascular retina (asterisks). (BW: birth weight; GA: gestational age; OU: both eyes; PMA: postmenstrual age; UWF: ultra-wide field)

■ HYBRID RETINOPATHY OF PREMATURITY

Human fetal retinal vascularization occurs from two distinct processes, that are: (1) vasculogenesis and (2) angiogenesis. Vasculogenesis involves formation of primordial vascular arcades of the superficial vascular plexus that is centered at the optic nerve head followed by angiogenesis which ends when the superficial and deeper retinal plexus reaches the ora serrata. Angiogenesis is driven by hypoxia-induced VEGF 165 which is responsible for more sever aggressive posterior ROP; vasculogenesis, which is independent of hypoxia-induced VEGF 165, is responsible for peripheral staged ROP. Hybrid ROP occurs whenever there is overlapping involvement of both vasculogenesis and angiogenesis. These eyes will have features of both A-ROP with abnormal neovascularization mainly involving posterior pole and features of classical staged ROP.[3]

■ BOTH EYES HYBRID RETINOPATHY OF PREMATURITY

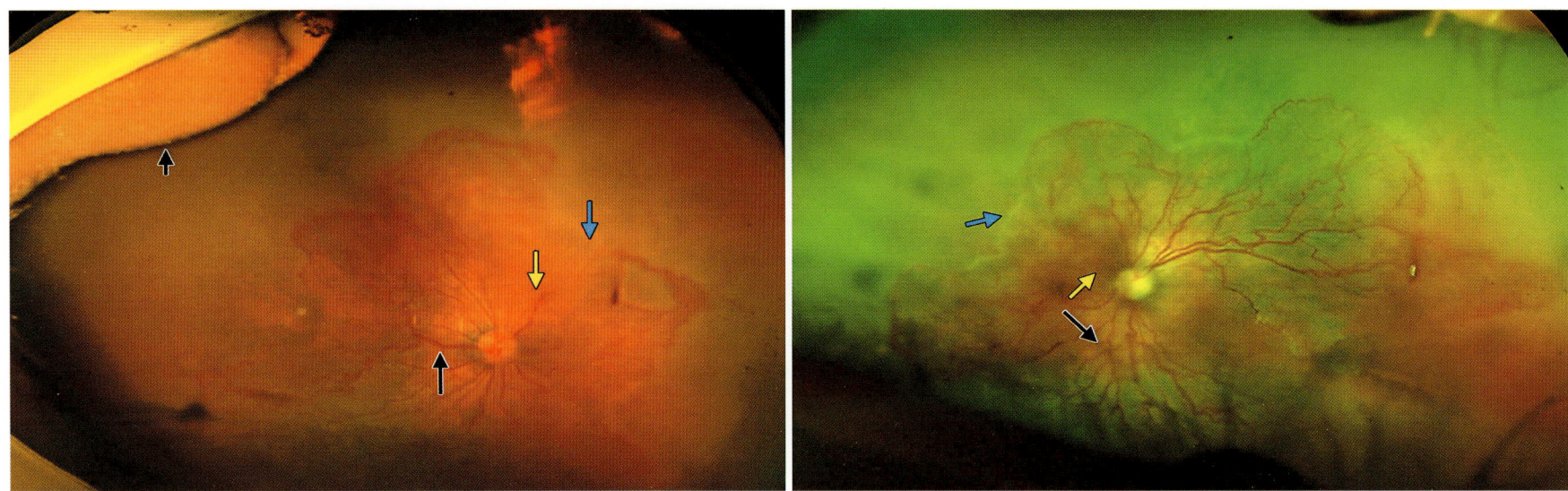

Fig. 2: UWF fundus photos of OU of 36 weeks PMA baby with 32 weeks GA and 1,350 g BW showing tortuous posterior vessels (black arrow) and new vessel fronds (yellow arrow) in posterior pole along with stage 2 in zone II posterior (blue arrow). Both the eyes needed laser photocoagulation. OD image (left) shows nose artifact (black short arrow). (BW: birth weight; GA: gestational age; OU: both eyes; PMA: postmenstrual age; UWF: ultra-wide field)

RETINOPATHY OF PREMATURITY WITH EXUDATION

Retinopathy of prematurity can rarely present with exudative detachment as an initial presentation.[4,5] It can be due severe hypoxia with poor scaffolding for retinal angiogenesis and poor blood retinal barrier leading to significant plasma leakage and exudation.[6] It can also occur secondary to inflammation following extensive laser photocoagulation treatment.[4,5] Clinically, fundus shows subretinal exudation, exudates along the dilated and tortuous blood vessels and retinal edema. Neonatal endophthalmitis and viral retinitis can be one of the vital differentials. Antivascular endothelial growth factor therapy or laser photocoagulation or a combination of both can be consider as treatment options.

BOTH EYES AGGRESSIVE RETINOPATHY OF PREMATURITY WITH EXUDATION AT INITIAL PRESENTATION

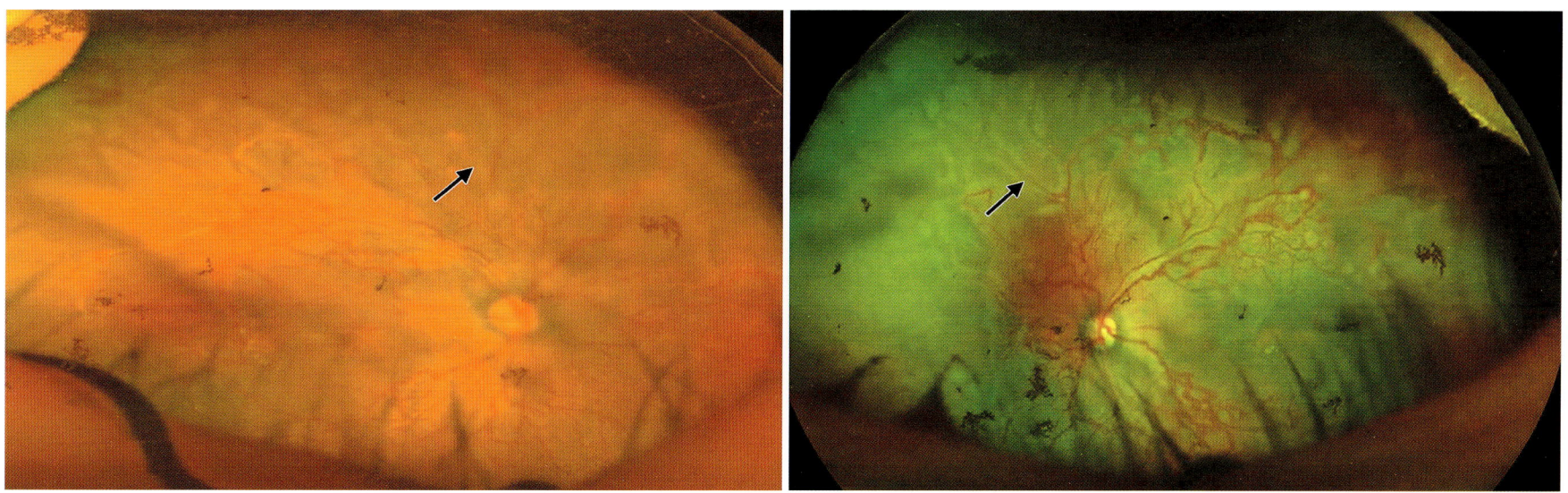

Fig. 3: UWF fundus photos of OU of 34 weeks PMA baby with 30 weeks GA and 1,700 g BW with extensive dilatation and tortuosity of posterior vessel and beyond along with diffuse shallow exudative detachment and exudation along the tortuous vessels (black arrow). (BW: birth weight; GA: gestational age; OU: both eyes; PMA: postmenstrual age; UWF: ultra-wide field)

■ BOTH EYES EXUDATIVE DETACHMENT AS INITIAL PRESENTATION IN AGGRESSIVE RETINOPATHY OF PREMATURITY

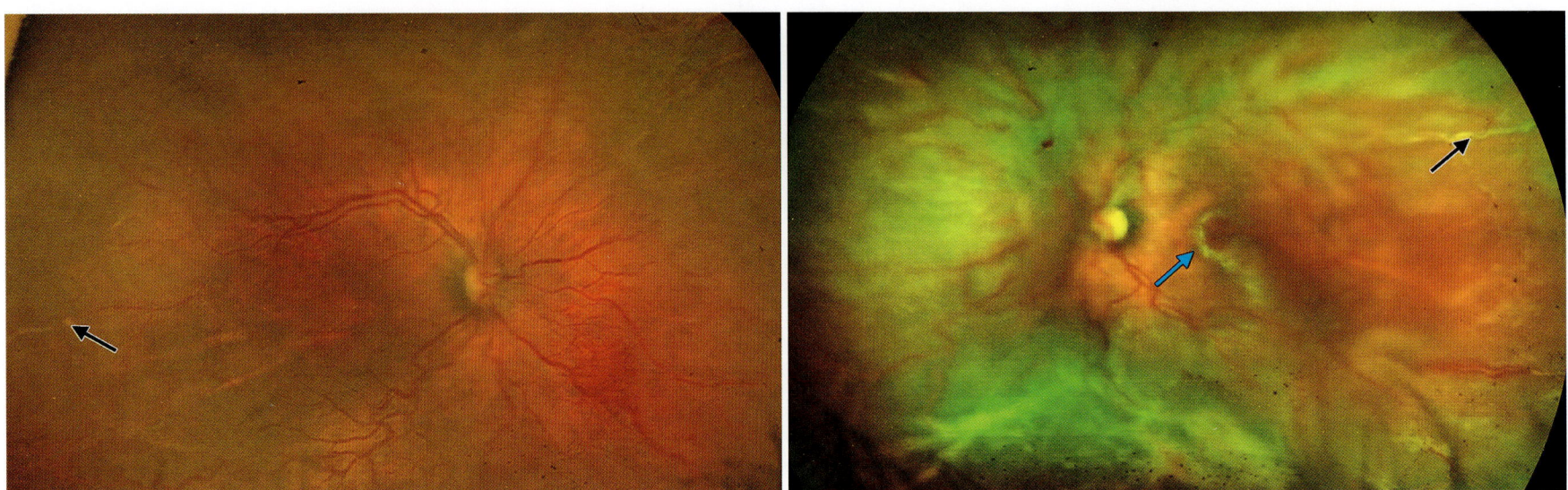

Fig. 4: UWF fundus photos of OU 30 weeks PMA baby with 28 weeks GA and 1,100 g BW with severe dilatation and tortuosity of vessels along with exudative detachment (OS more than OD), exudation along the vessels (black arrow) and at the fovea (blue arrow). (BW: birth weight; GA: gestational age; OD: right eye; OS: left eye; OU: both eyes; PMA: postmenstrual age; UWF: ultra-wide field)

■ REFERENCES

1. Chiang MF, Quinn GE, Fielder AR, Ostmo SR, Paul Chan RV, Berrocal A, et al. International Classification of Retinopathy of Prematurity, Third Edition. Ophthalmology. 2021;128(10):e51-e68.
2. Flynn JT, Chan-Ling T. Retinopathy of prematurity: two distinct mechanisms that underlie zone 1 and zone 2 disease. Am J Ophthalmol. 2006;142(1):46-59.
3. Sanghi G, Dogra MR, Dogra M, Katoch D, Gupta A. A hybrid form of retinopathy of prematurity. Br J Ophthalmol. 2012;96(4):519-22.
4. Jayanna S, Agarwal K, Padhi TR, Jalali S. Exudative retinal detachment as an initial presentation in retinopathy of prematurity. J AAPOS. 2020;24(6):374-6.
5. Agarwal K, Jayanna S, Padhi TR, Jalali S. Exudative retinal detachment as an initial presentation of retinopathy of prematurity: Clinical profile and outcomes of a rare presentation. Indian J Ophthalmol. 2022;70(7):2486-9.
6. Hartnett ME. Pathophysiology and mechanisms of severe retinopathy of prematurity. Ophthalmology. 2015;122(1):200-10.

Interventions and Follow-up in Retinopathy of Prematurity

INTRODUCTION

Retinopathy of prematurity (ROP) warranting immediate treatment is subgrouped as type 1 ROP. Laser photocoagulation and intravitreal antivascular endothelial growth factor (anti-VEGF) injections are the two major treatment strategies at present, except for stages 4 and 5 where additional surgical intervention is required. This chapter depicts various interventions and its responses during follow-up visits. Type 2 ROP can be closely observed. Type 1 ROP requires active intervention such as retinal laser, intravitreal anti-VEGF, surgery, either alone or in combination.

LASER PHOTOCOAGULATION IN ROP

Laser photocoagualtion is still the gold standered treatment for ROP. A head-worn indirect laser system is the most convenient to treat the babies in lying posture. Laser is useful in type 1 ROP which includes aggressive retinopathy of prematurity (A-ROP), any stage of ROP with plus disease; stage 3 ROP without plus disease, and zone II, stage 2 or 3 ROP with plus disease. Either diode red (810 nm) or double frequency Nd-Yag green (532 nm) laser is used.[1,2]

It can be safely done under topical anesthesia under careful monitoring of the vitals and services of neonatal intensive care and anesthetist. Adequate number of laser spots in avascular retina and 2–3 rows posterior to the ridge in staged ROP is recommended. Extensively confluent laser spots can cause exudative detachments, hypotony, and cataract. Signs of regression includes clearing of retinal/preretinal and vitreous hemorrhages, regression of dilatation and tortuosity of retinal vessels.[1]

ANTIVASCULAR ENDOTHELIAL GROWTH FACTOR THERAPY IN ROP

Antivascular endothelial growth factor therapy is the treatment of choice in A-ROP with hazy media, nondilating pupil and in poorly developed vascularity in macular region. It can also be used in staged ROP with plus disease[3] provided there is no active traction. Commonly used anti-VEGF in ROP are bevacizumab (BEAT ROP study) and ranibizumab (RAINBOW study); in either case one-third of the adult dose is used.[4] Signs of regression are clearing of media, and reduced tortuosity of vessels, seen within a week of treatment. Peripheral retina in such cases may remain avascular for longer time and hence requires closer and longer follow-up as recurrence can occur, more often after anti-VEGF monotherapy.

SURGERY IN ROP

Pars plana vitrectomy is indicated in stage 4a and 4b with tractional retinal detachments. It can be combined with retinal laser or anti-VEGF intravitreal injection preoperatively to reduce the severity. In stage 5 ROP, pars plana lensectomy is usually required. The surgical anatomy of infant's eye is different from adult eye; it is a small eye with steeper cornea, short axial length, less tensile sclera and densely adherent vitreous. These features must be considered during the procedure. Other indication of surgery in ROP includes nonresolving dense vitreous hemorrhages and rhegmatogenous retinal detachments. Scleral buckle can also be considered in cases of rhegmatogenous detachment. Good surgical outcome includes falling back of retinal fold with no active traction in cases of stage 4 and opening of the funnel with visibility of disc in stage 5 ROP.[5,6]

■ BOTH EYES REGRESSING STAGE 2, ZONE II, PLUS AFTER 2 WEEKS OF LASER

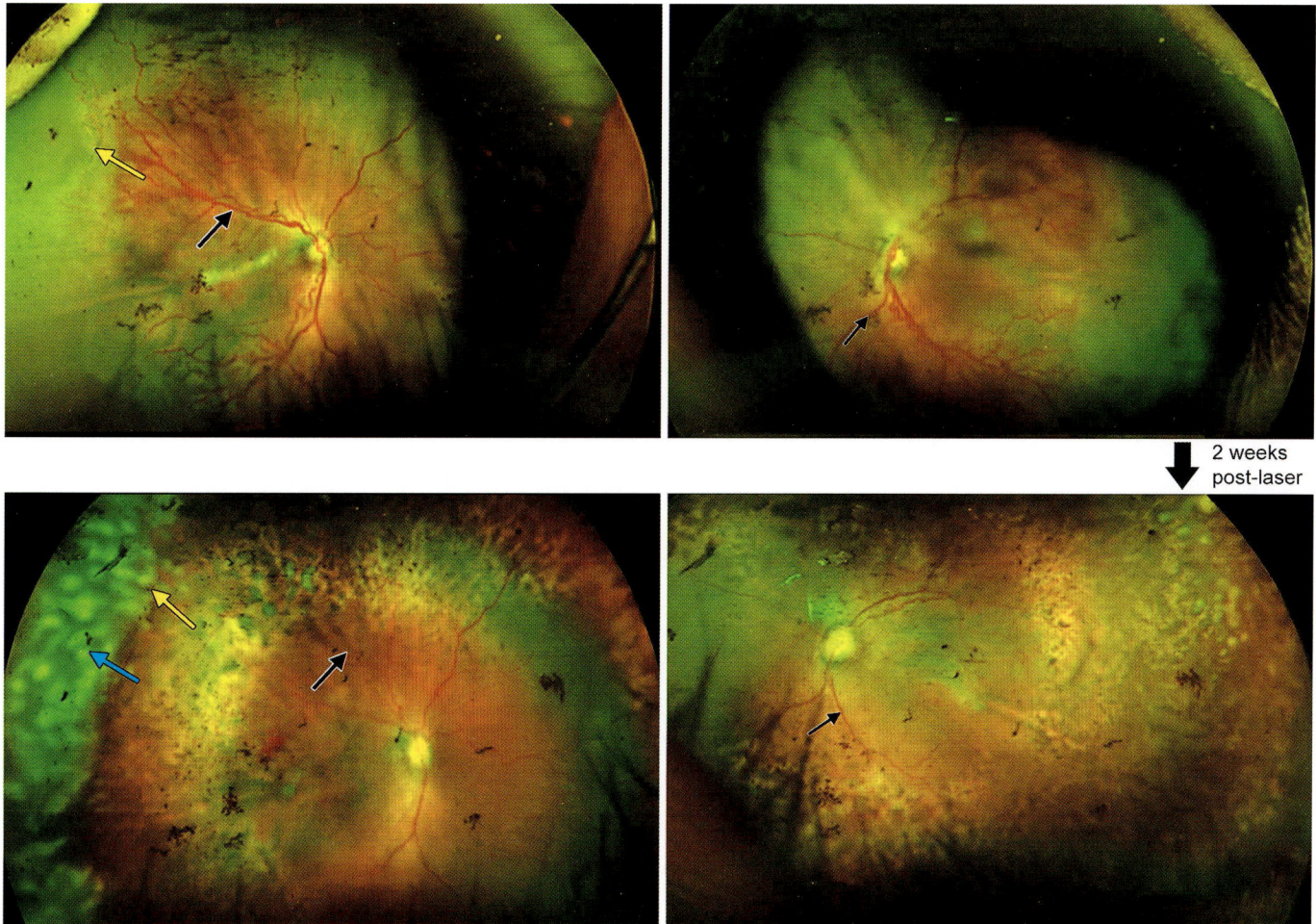

Fig. 1: UWF fundus of OU of 38 weeks PMA baby with 26 weeks GA and 1,400 g BW with type 1 ROP, stage 2, zone II plus (upper panel) regressed well, 2 weeks after laser photocoagulation (lower panel) characterized by reduced tortuosity (black arrow), disappearance of ridge (yellow arrow), and fresh laser marks (blue arrow) in the lower panel images. (BW: birth weight; GA: gestational age; OU: both eyes; PMA: postmenstrual age; ROP: aggressive retinopathy of prematurity; UWF: ultra-wide field)

■ BOTH EYES REGRESSING AGGRESSIVE ROP 2 MONTHS AFTER LASER

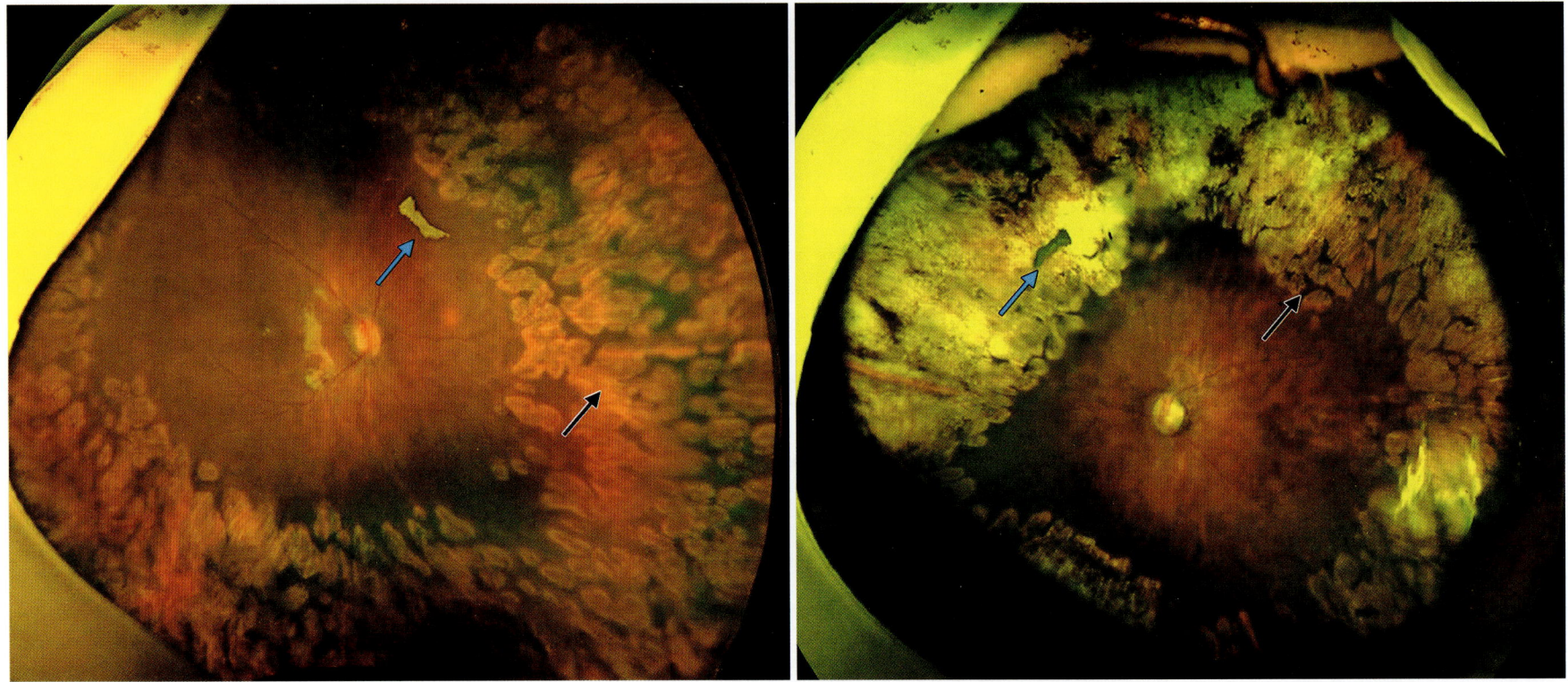

Fig. 2: UWF fundus images of OU of 36 weeks PMA baby with 30 weeks GA, and 1,400 g BW with well regressed A-ROP, 2 months after laser photocoagulation. Extensive coalesced laser marks in zone II and III (black arrow) are seen and the vessel tortuosity is disappeared. A reflection artefact of a foreign material on the camera lens can be seen in both eyes (blue arrow). (A-ROP: aggressive retinopathy of prematurity; BW: birth weight; GA: gestational age; OU: both eyes; PMA: postmenstrual age; UWF: ultra-wide field)

■ BOTH EYES REGRESSING STAGE 4A ROP, 1 WEEK AFTER LASER

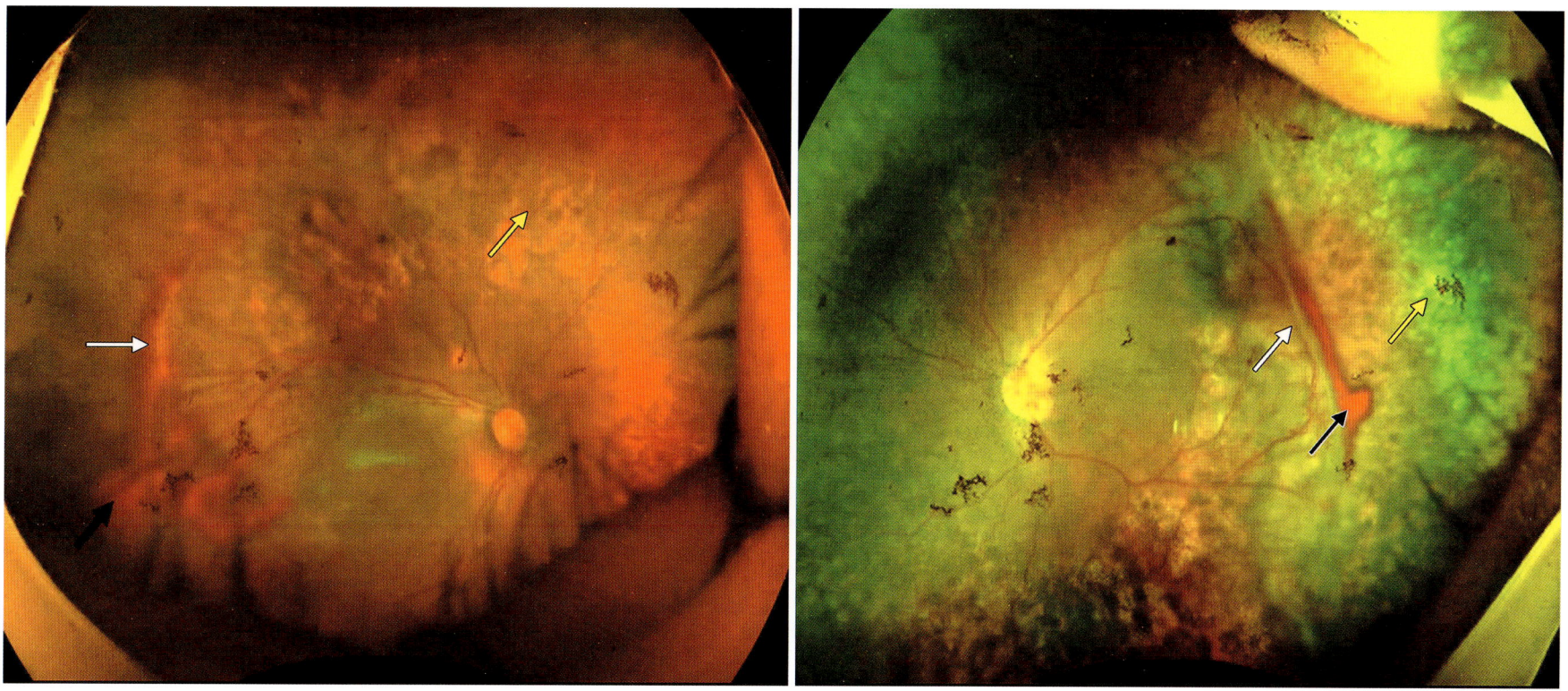

Fig. 3: UWF fundus images of OU of 41 weeks PMA baby with 30 weeks GA, and 1,100 g BW with regressing ridge with no active traction (white arrow) and residual hemorrhage (black arrow) 1 week after laser treatment; laser marks are seen (yellow arrow). (BW: birth weight; GA: gestational age; OU: both eyes; PMA: postmenstrual age; UWF: ultra-wide field)

BOTH EYES ANTERIOR LASER SKIP AREAS IN ZONE III STAGE 3 ROP

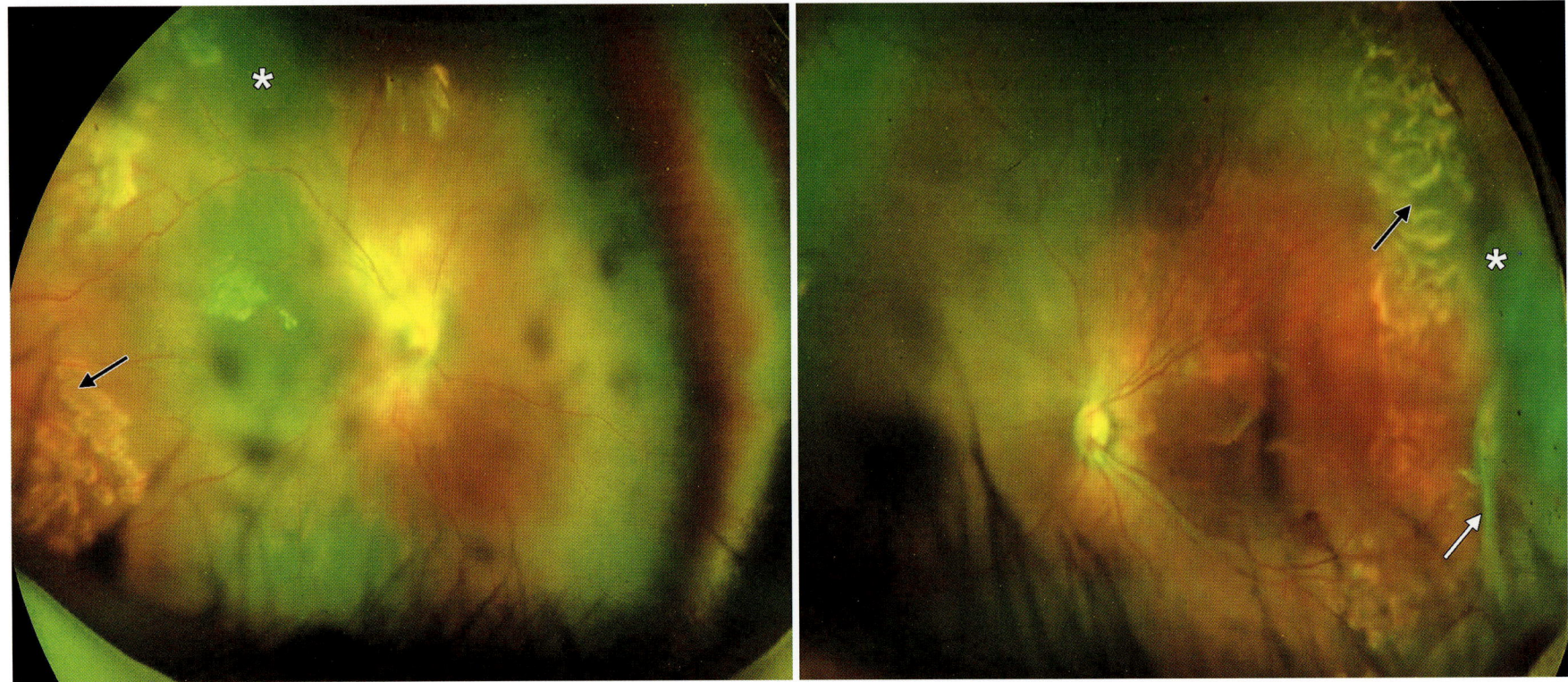

Fig. 4: UWF fundus images of OU of 34 weeks PMA baby with 28 weeks GA, and 1,200 g BW showing persistent, tortuosity of vessels elevate ridge (white arrow) with scanty laser marks (black arrow) and extensive skip areas (asterisks). (BW: birth weight; GA: gestational age; OU: both eyes; PMA: postmenstrual age; UWF: ultra-wide field)

BOTH EYES SKIP LASER AREAS IN NONREGRESSING AGGRESSIVE ROP WITH PRERETINAL HEMORRHAGE PROGRESSING TO STAGE 4A ROP

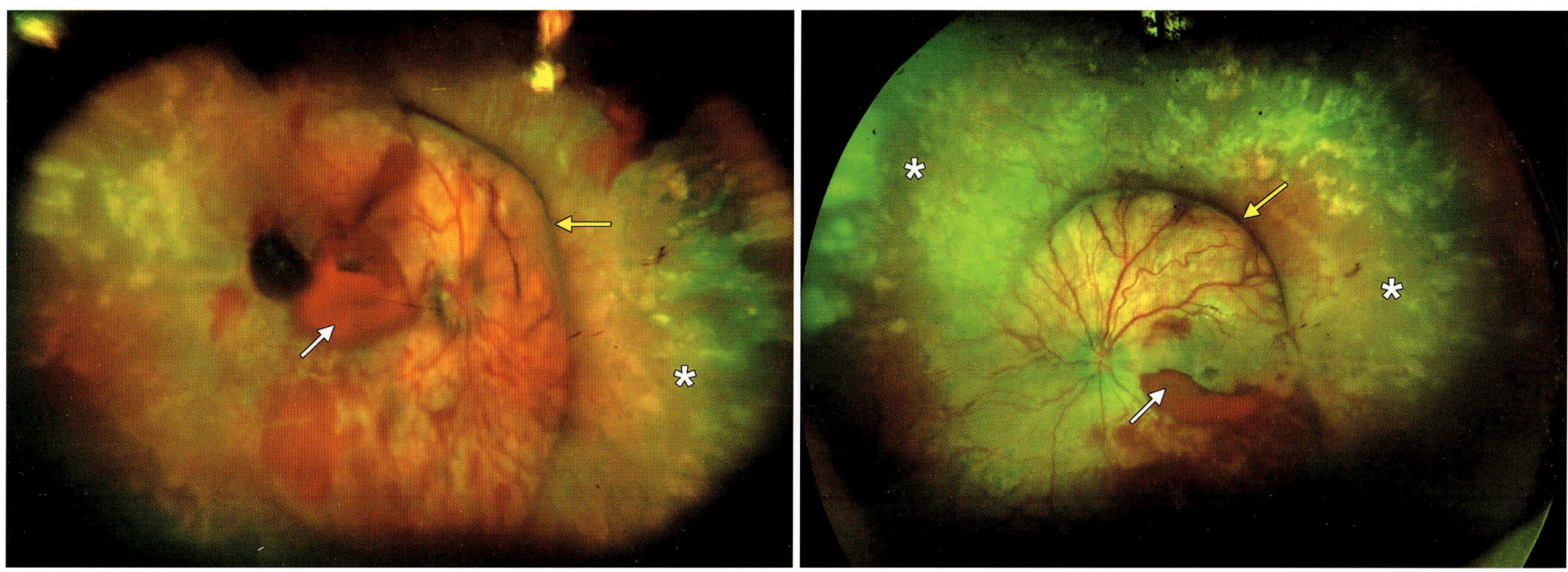

Fig. 5: UWF fundus images of OU of 40 weeks PMA baby with 33 weeks GA and 1,100 g BW showing persistent tortuosity of vessel, vitreous hemorrhage (white arrow) and elevated retina along with ridge (yellow arrow) due to inadequate laser photocoagulation with skip areas (asterisks). (BW: birth weight; GA: gestational age; OU: both eyes; PMA: postmenstrual age; UWF: ultra-wide field)

BOTH EYES EXUDATIVE RETINAL DETACHMENT AFTER EXTENSIVE LASER, RESOLVED AFTER 1 MONTH OF TOPICAL STEROIDS AND CYCLOPLEGICS

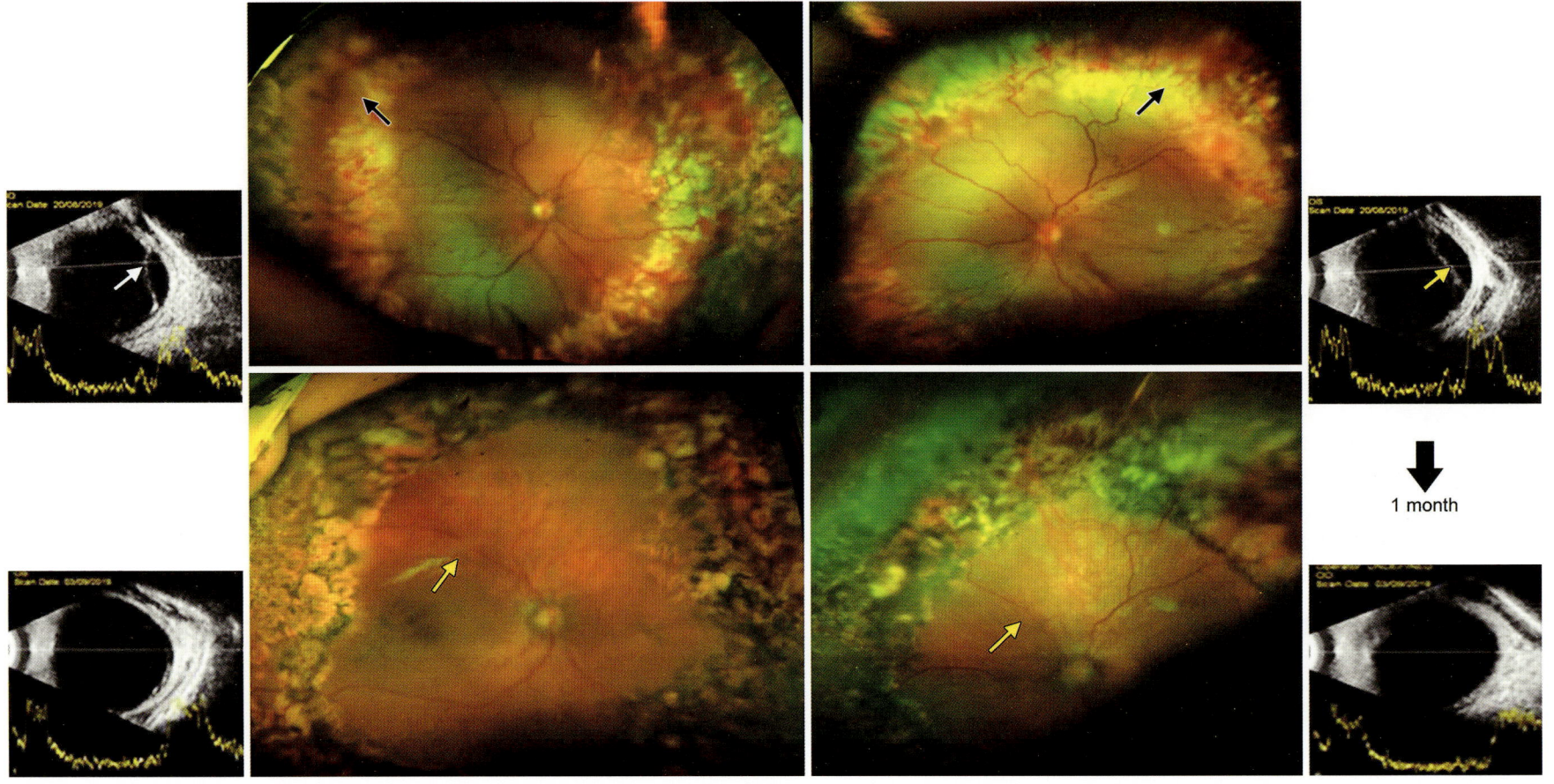

Fig. 6: UWF fundus images of OU of 38 weeks PMA baby with 25 weeks GA and 700 g BW.

Notes:
Upper panel: Diffuse exudative detachment confirmed on B-scan (white arrow) secondary to extensive laser (black arrow).
Lower panel: Retinal detachment resolved after 1 month of treatment with topical steroids and cycloplegics, confirmed on B-scan and regressed tortuosity of vessels (yellow arrow).
(BW: birth weight; GA: gestational age; OU: both eyes; PMA: postmenstrual age; UWF: ultra-wide field)

BOTH EYES REGRESSING AGGRESSIVE ROP WITH RESOLVING PRERETINAL HEMORRHAGE 1 WEEK AFTER INTRAVITREAL BEVACIZUMAB

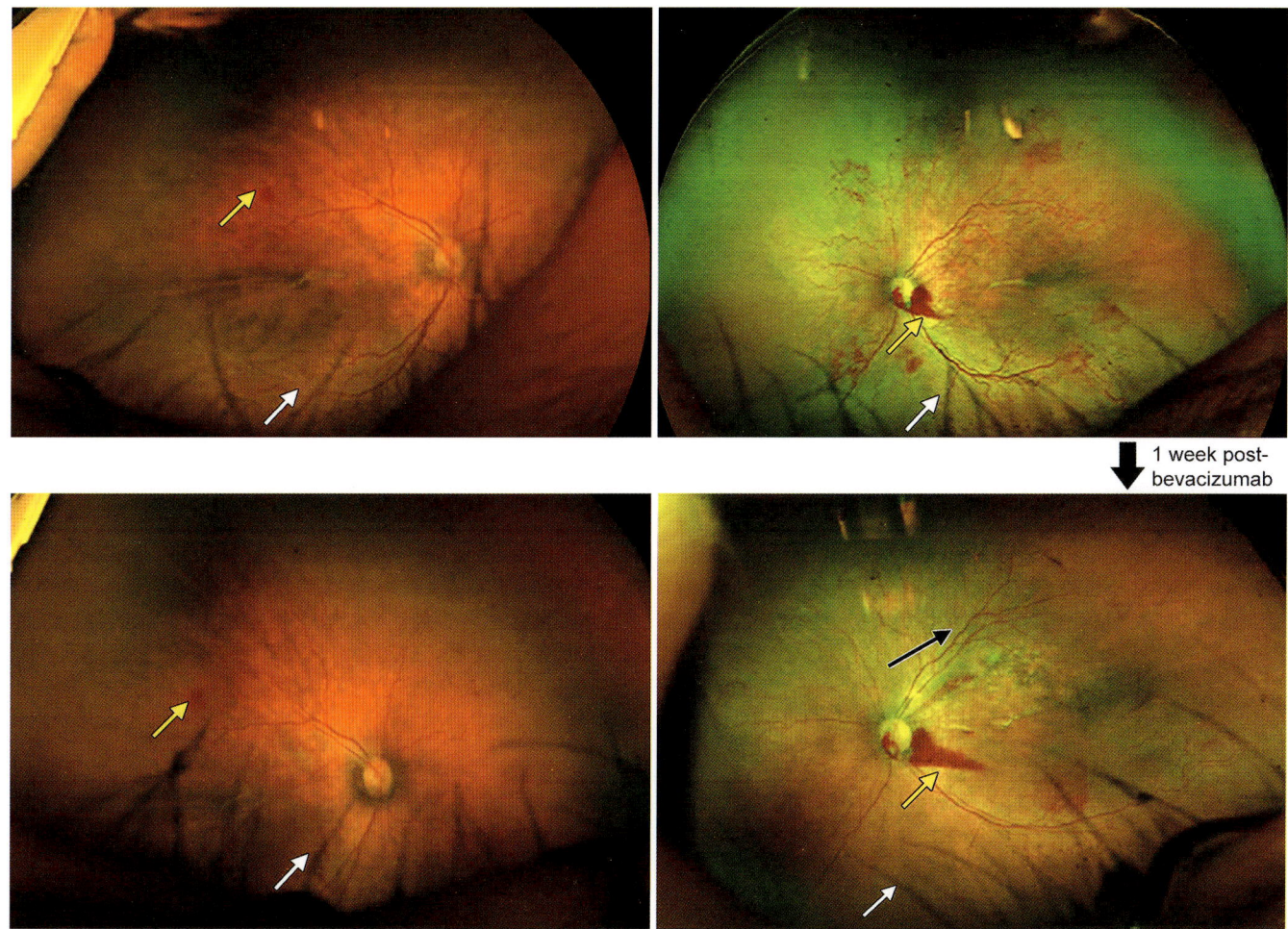

Fig. 7: UWF fundus images of OU of 33 weeks PMA baby with 30 weeks GA and 1,300 g BW.
Notes:
Upper panel: OU had aggressive ROP and OS had preretinal hemorrhages (yellow arrow).
Lower panel: Regressing ROP characterized with reduced tortuosity of vessels (black arrow) 1 week after treating with intravitreal bevacizumab. Eye lash artefacts are seen in all images (white arrow).
(BW: birth weight; GA: gestational age; OU: both eyes; OS: left eye; PMA: postmenstrual age; ROP: retinopathy of prematurity; UWF: ultra-wide field)

BOTH EYES ZONE III AVASCULAR RETINA, 3 MONTHS AFTER INTRAVITREAL BEVACIZUMAB INJECTION IN AGGRESSIVE ROP

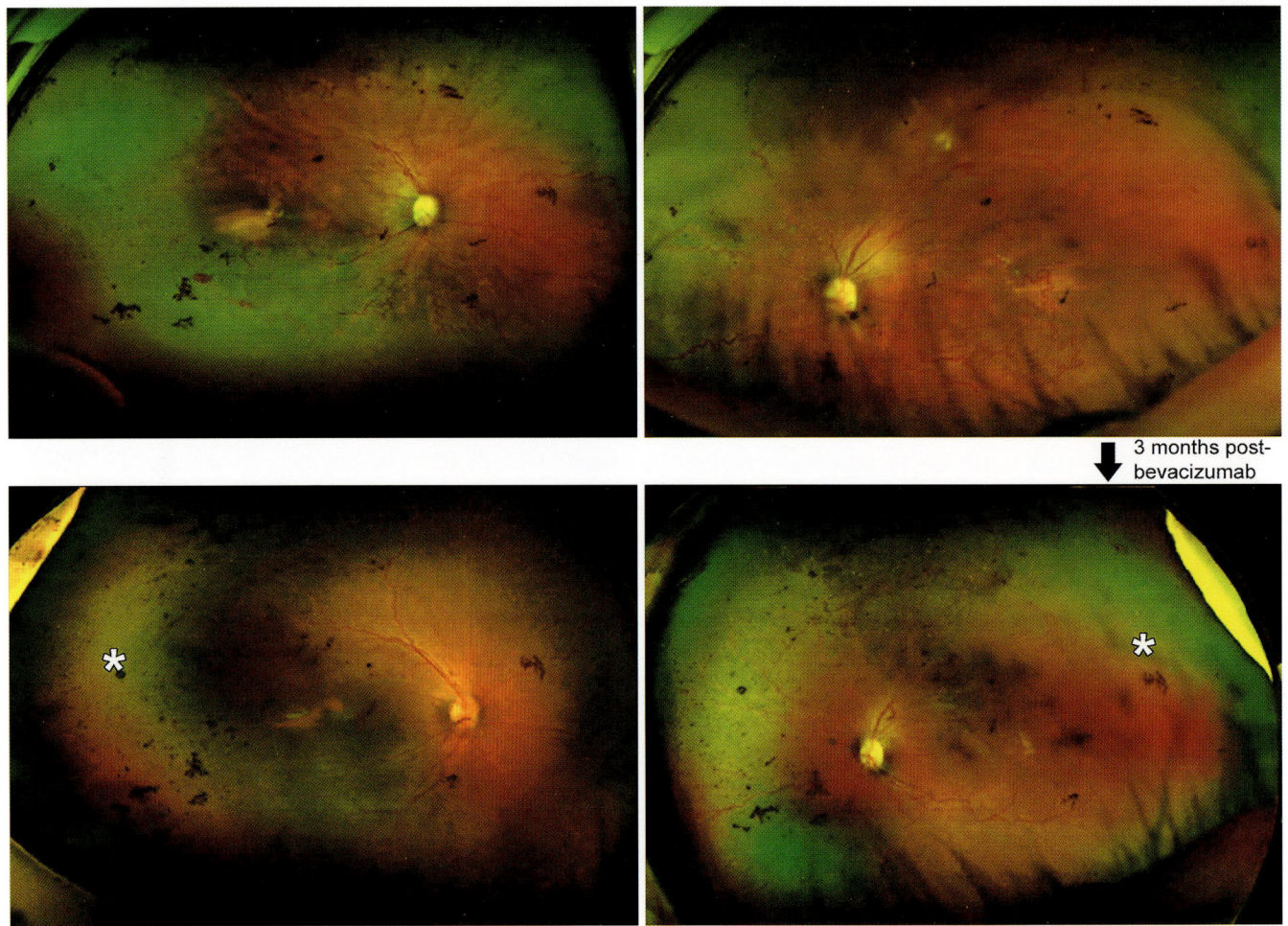

Fig. 8: UWF fundus images of OU of 36 weeks PMA baby with 30 weeks GA and 1,100 g BW with upper panel—aggressive ROP OU and lower panel—complete regression in 3 months; persistence of avascular zone in zone III can be seen (asterisks). (BW: birth weight; GA: gestational age; OU: both eyes; PMA: postmenstrual age; ROP: retinopathy of prematurity; UWF: ultra-wide field)

LEFT EYE NONREGRESSING ROP AFTER 4 WEEKS OF INTRAVITREAL BEVACIZUMAB FOR BOTH EYES AGGRESSIVE ROP

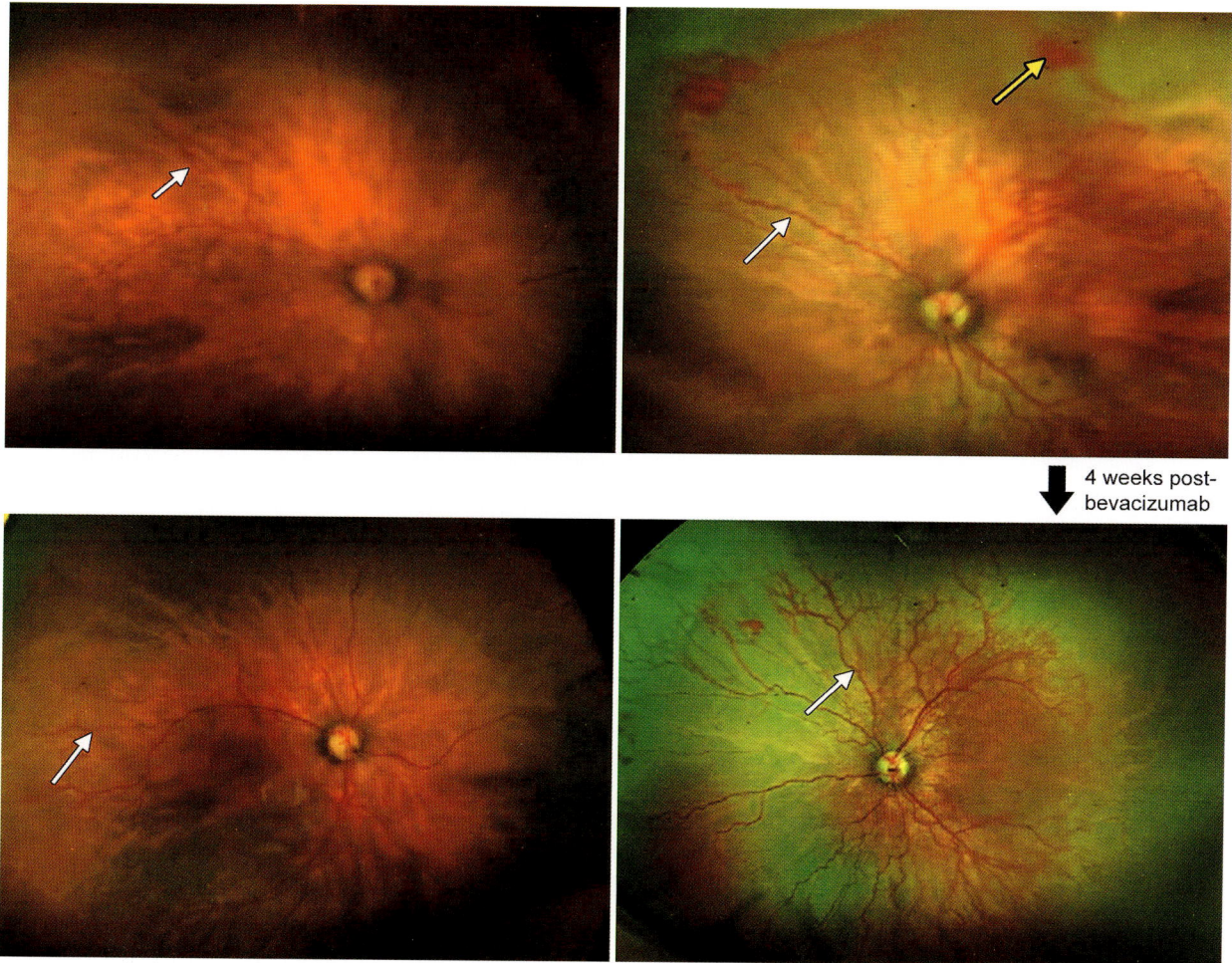

Fig. 9: UWF fundus images of OU of 36 weeks PMA baby with 31 weeks GA and 1,400 g BW.
Notes:
Upper panel: OU A-ROP and OS preretinal hemorrhages (yellow arrow). OU treated with intravitreal bevacizumab.
Lower panel: No signs of regression 4 weeks after intravitreal bevacizumab. Persistent tortuosity of posterior pole vessels and beyond is seen (white arrow).
(A-ROP: aggressive retinopathy of prematurity; BW: birth weight; GA: gestational age; OU: both eyes; OS: left eye; PMA: postmenstrual age; UWF: ultra-wide field)

■ AGGRESSIVE ROP IN TRIPLET REGRESSING 1 WEEK AFTER INTRAVITREAL BEVACIZUMAB

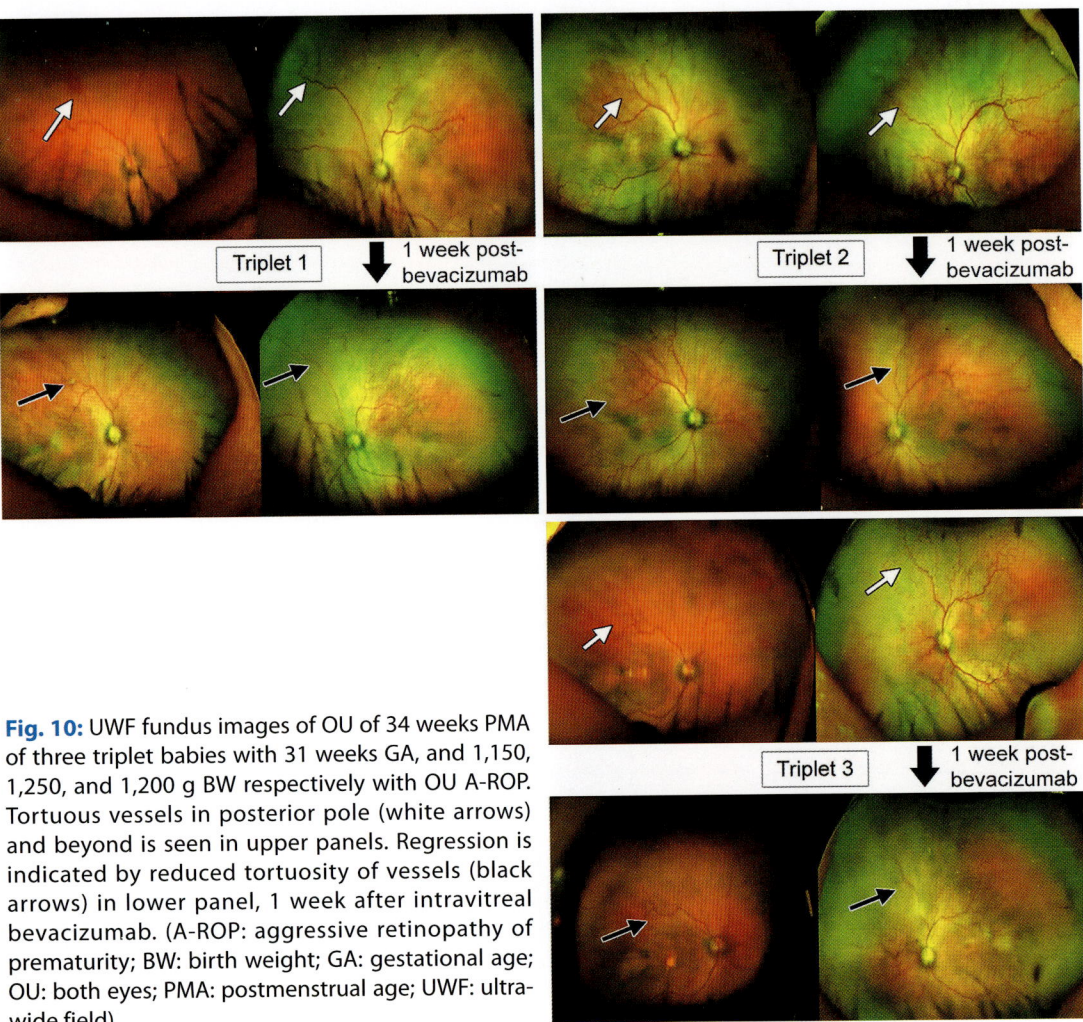

Fig. 10: UWF fundus images of OU of 34 weeks PMA of three triplet babies with 31 weeks GA, and 1,150, 1,250, and 1,200 g BW respectively with OU A-ROP. Tortuous vessels in posterior pole (white arrows) and beyond is seen in upper panels. Regression is indicated by reduced tortuosity of vessels (black arrows) in lower panel, 1 week after intravitreal bevacizumab. (A-ROP: aggressive retinopathy of prematurity; BW: birth weight; GA: gestational age; OU: both eyes; PMA: postmenstrual age; UWF: ultra-wide field)

■ BOTH EYES AGGRESSIVE ROP REGRESSING TO STAGE 2 IN LEFT EYE, 2 WEEKS AFTER INTRAVITREAL BEVACIZUMAB

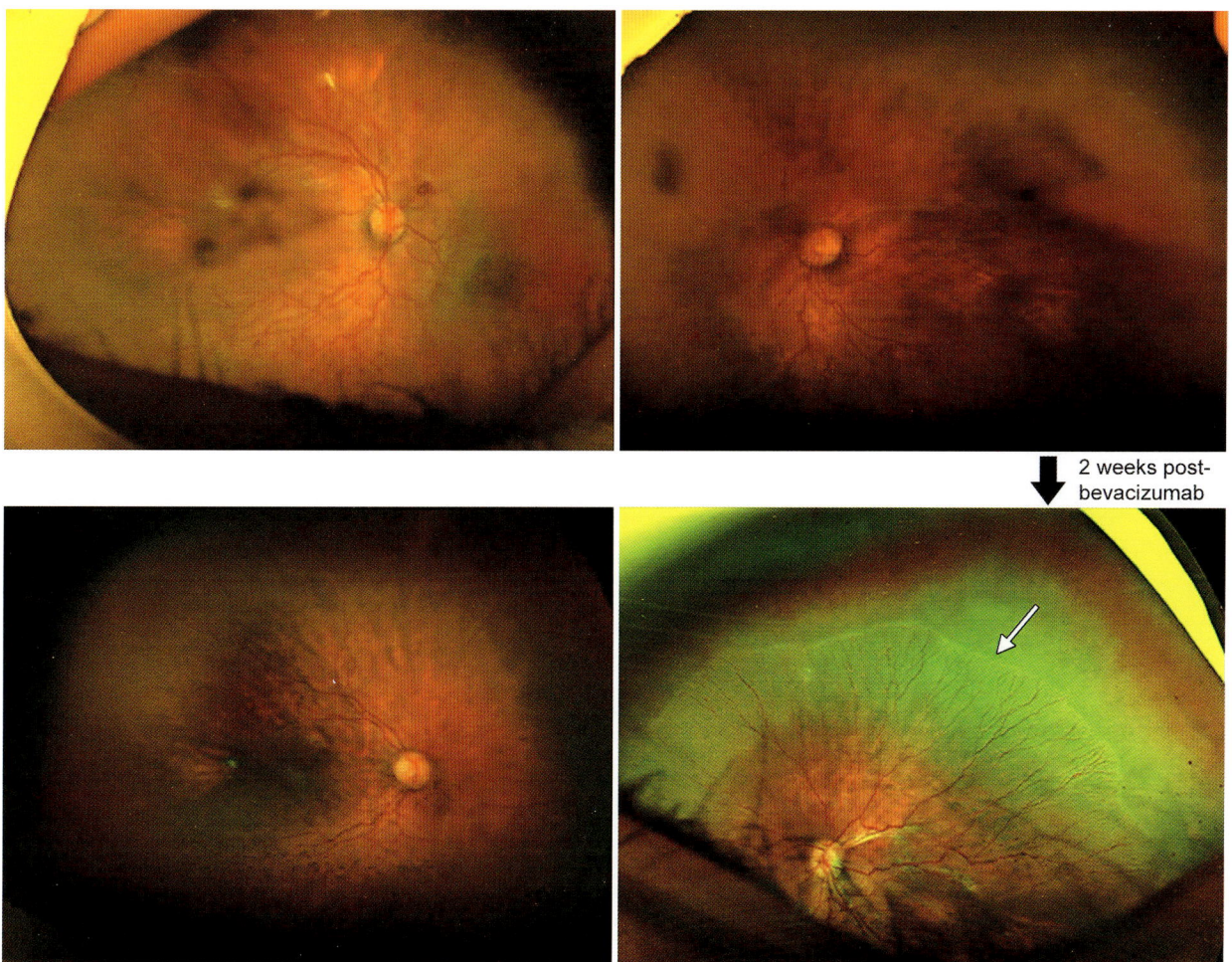

Fig. 11: UWF fundus images of OU of 36 weeks PMA baby with 28 weeks GA and 1,200 g BW. A-ROP (upper panel) developed flat ridge in OS (white arrow) along with regression of tortuous vessels (lower panel) 2 weeks after intravitreal bevacizumab (one-third of the adult dose). (A-ROP: aggressive retinopathy of prematurity; BW: birth weight; GA: gestational age; OU: both eyes; OS: left eye; PMA: postmenstrual age; UWF: ultra-wide field)

■ REGRESSING AGGRESSIVE ROP WITH EXUDATION 1 WEEK AFTER INTRAVITREAL BEVACIZUMAB INJECTION

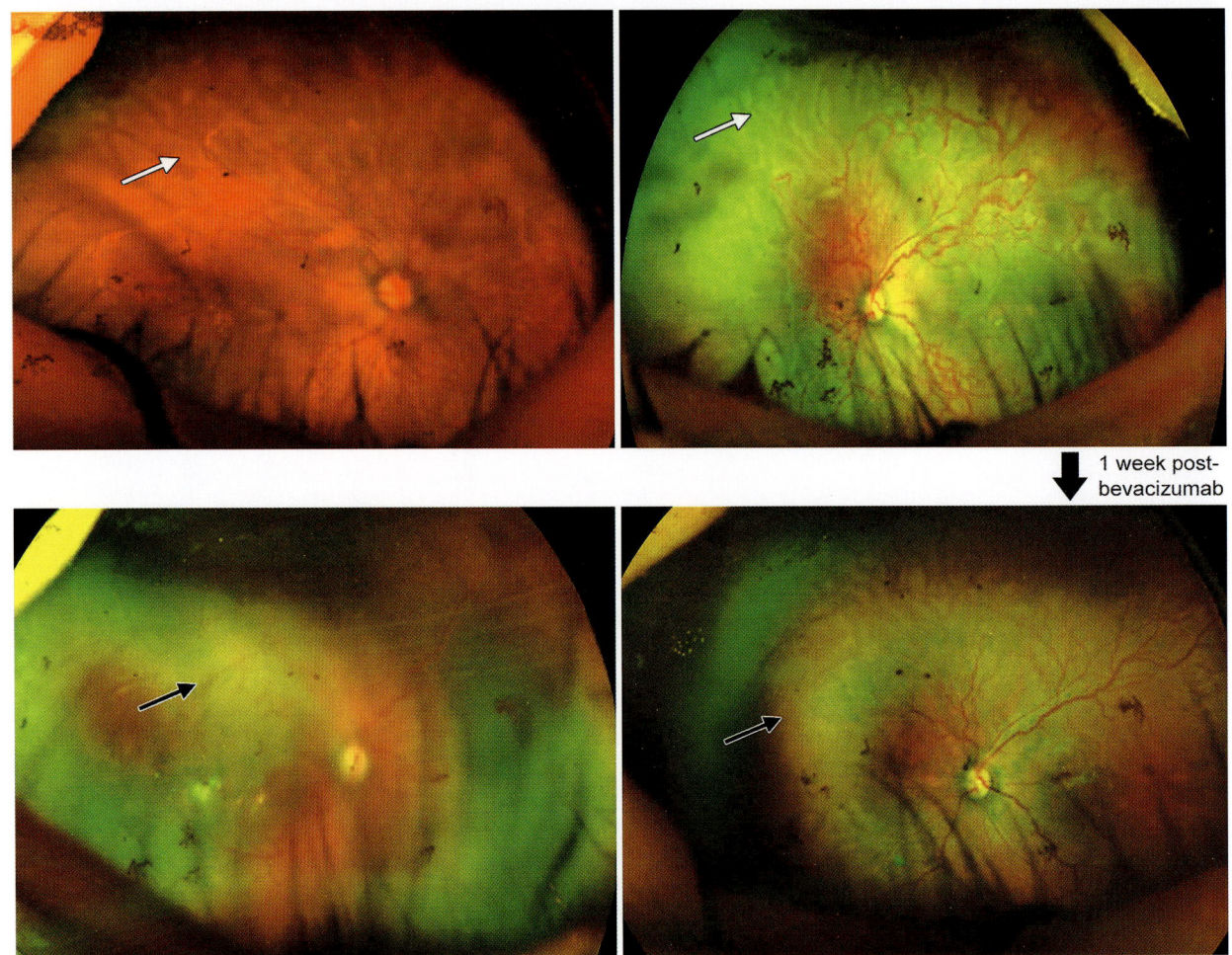

Fig. 12: UWF fundus images of OU of 34 weeks PMA baby with 30 weeks GA, and 1,700 g BW with A-ROP and exudative detachment and exudates along the vessels (white arrows, upper panel). Disease regression 1 week after intravitreal bevacizumab with exudation resolved and vessel tortuosity reduced (black arrows, lower panel). (A-ROP: aggressive retinopathy of prematurity; BW: birth weight; GA: gestational age; OU: both eyes; PMA: postmenstrual age; UWF: ultra-wide field)

BOTH EYES REGRESSING AGGRESSIVE ROP AFTER COMBINATION TREATMENT

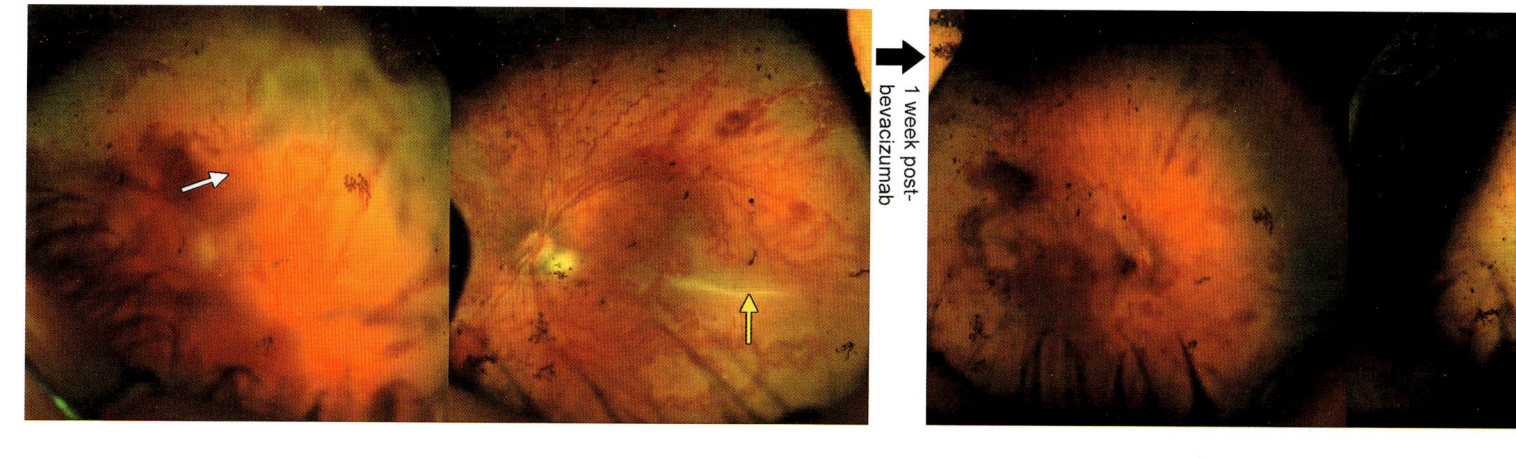

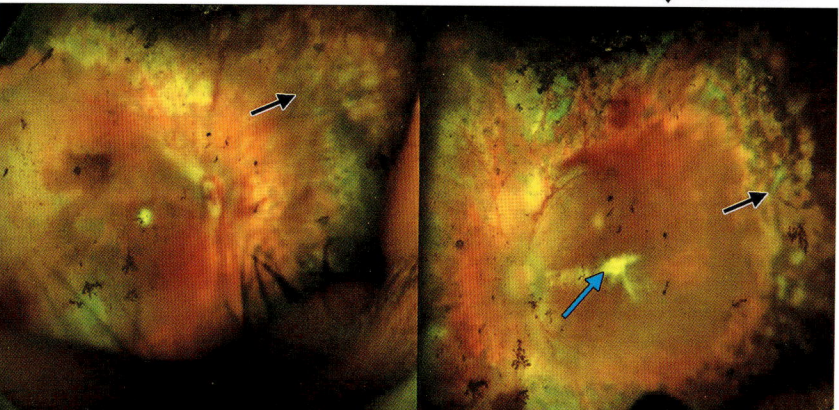

Fig. 13: UWF fundus images of OU of 34 weeks PMA baby with 28 weeks GA, and 1,200 g BW.
Notes:
Left panel: A-ROP—preretinal hemorrhages (white arrow) and exudation (yellow arrow).
Right panel: Reduced but persistent vessel tortuosity (top 1 week after intravitreal bevacizumab).
(A-ROP: aggressive retinopathy of prematurity; BW: birth weight; GA: gestational age; OU: both eyes; PMA: postmenstrual age; UWF: ultra-wide field)
Complete regression is seen 3 weeks after addition laser photocoagulation (bottom panel) adequate laser marks (black arrow) in periphery and epiretinal membrane (blue arrow) at fovea can also be seen.

■ BOTH EYES REGRESSING AGGRESSIVE ROP WITH EXUDATION AFTER COMBINATION TREATMENT

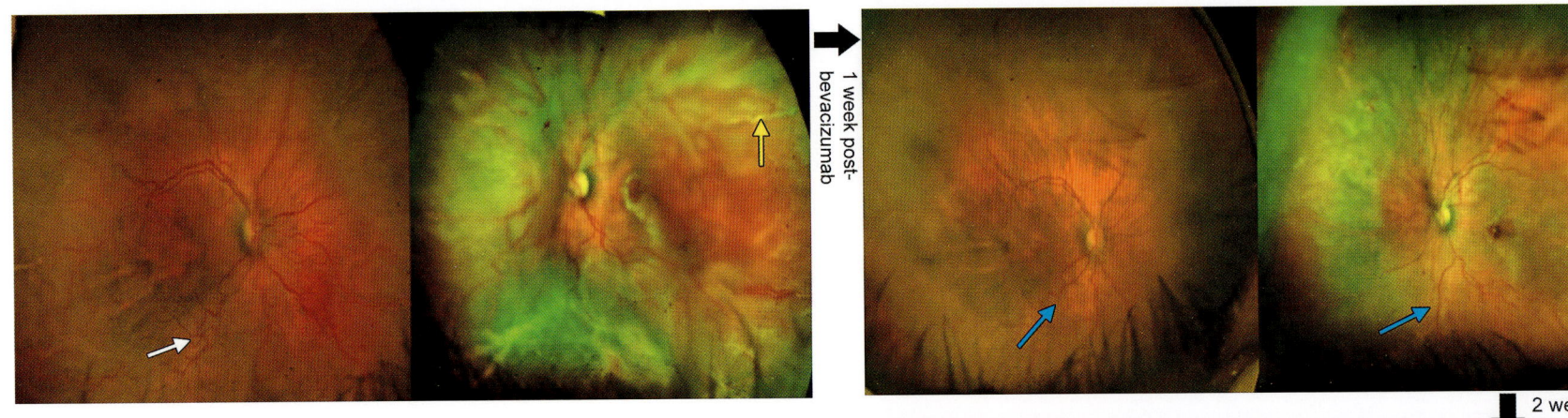

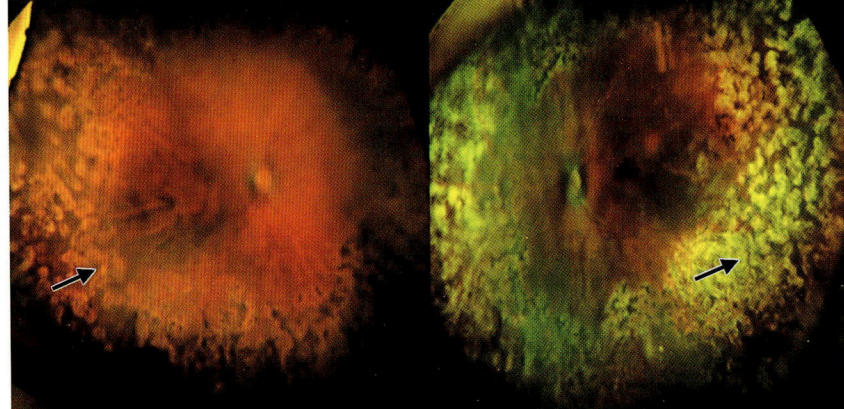

Fig. 14: UWF fundus images of OU of a 30 weeks PMA baby with 28 weeks GA and 1,100 g BW.

Notes:
Left panel: Both eyes had A-ROP, extensive tortuous vessels (white arrow), exudation along the vessels (yellow arrow), and exudative detachment.
Right panel: Resolved exudation, reduced but persistent vessel tortuosity (blue arrows in top). 1 week after intravitreal bevacizumab. Complete regression is seen 2 weeks after additional laser photocoagulation (bottom). Adequate laser marks (black arrow) in periphery is seen.
(A-ROP: aggressive retinopathy of prematurity; BW: birth weight; GA: gestational age; OU: both eyes; PMA: postmenstrual age; UWF: ultra-wide field)

■ RIGHT EYE RELIEVED TRACTION, 1 MONTH AFTER PARS PLANA VITRECTOMY IN STAGE 4 ROP

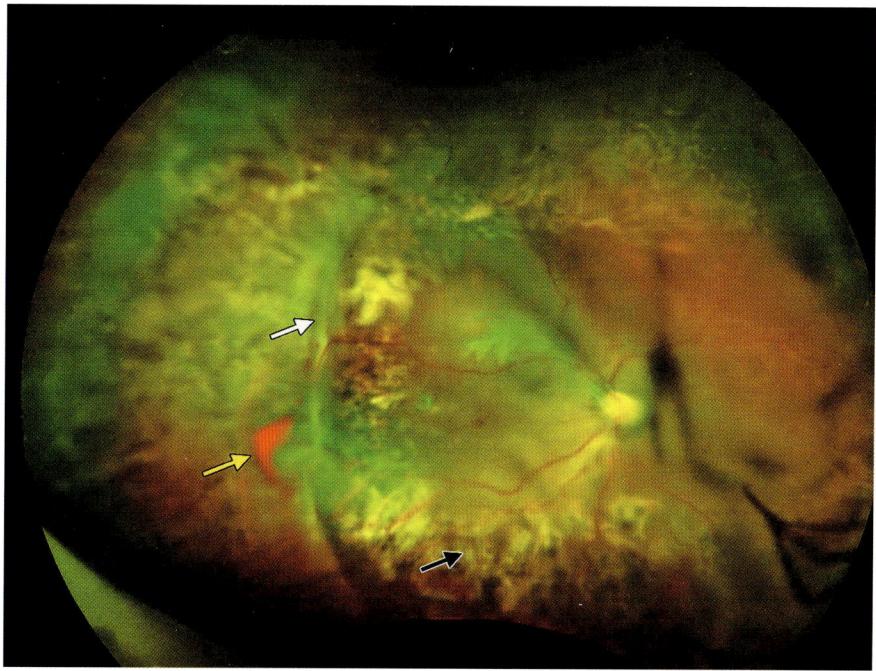

Fig. 15: UWF fundus images of OD of 36 weeks PMA baby with 28 weeks GA and 1,160 g BW. Notice temporal retinal fold free from traction (white arrow) seen 1 month after pars plana vitrectomy. Resolving preretinal hemorrhage (yellow arrow), adequate laser marks (black arrow) are seen. (BW: birth weight; GA: gestational age; OD: right eye; PMA: postmenstrual age; UWF: ultra-wide field)

■ BOTH EYES STAGE 2 FLAT RIDGE PROGRESS TO RIDGE DOUBLING IN 2 WEEKS

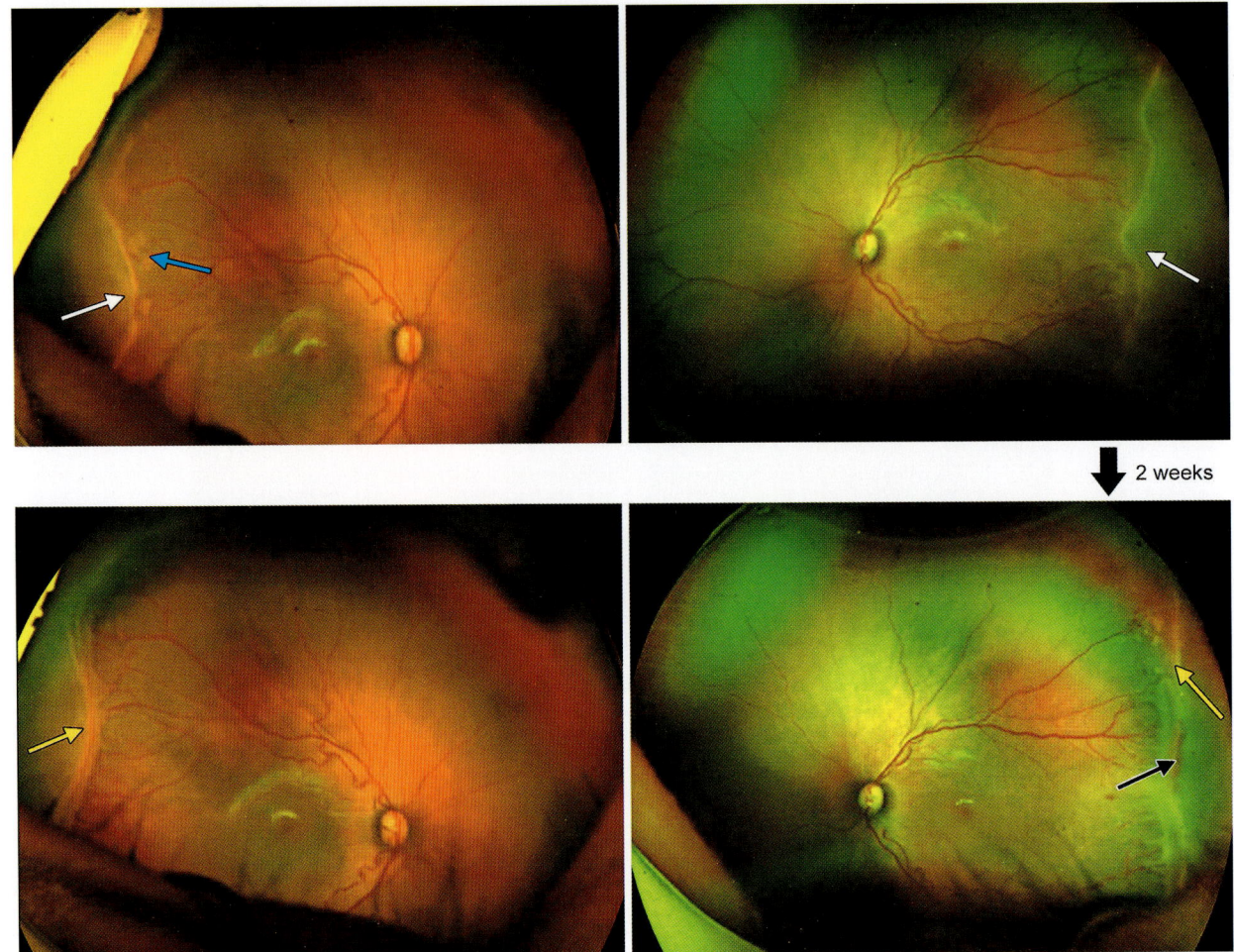

Fig. 16: UWF fundus images of OU of 34 weeks PMA baby with 29 weeks GA and 1,200 g BW.
Notes:
Upper panel: Stage 2 flat ridge (white arrows) zone II ROP with mild tortuosity of vessels.
Lower panel: Ridge doubling (yellow arrow) in 2 weeks follow up. Pop corn lesions (blue arrow) and hot dog-like linear hemorrhage (black arrow) are seen.
(BW: birth weight; GA: gestational age; OU: both eyes; PMA: postmenstrual age; ROP: retinopathy of prematurity; UWF: ultra-wide field)

■ NATURAL COURSE OF STAGED ROP-SELF REGRESSING TYPE 2 ROP

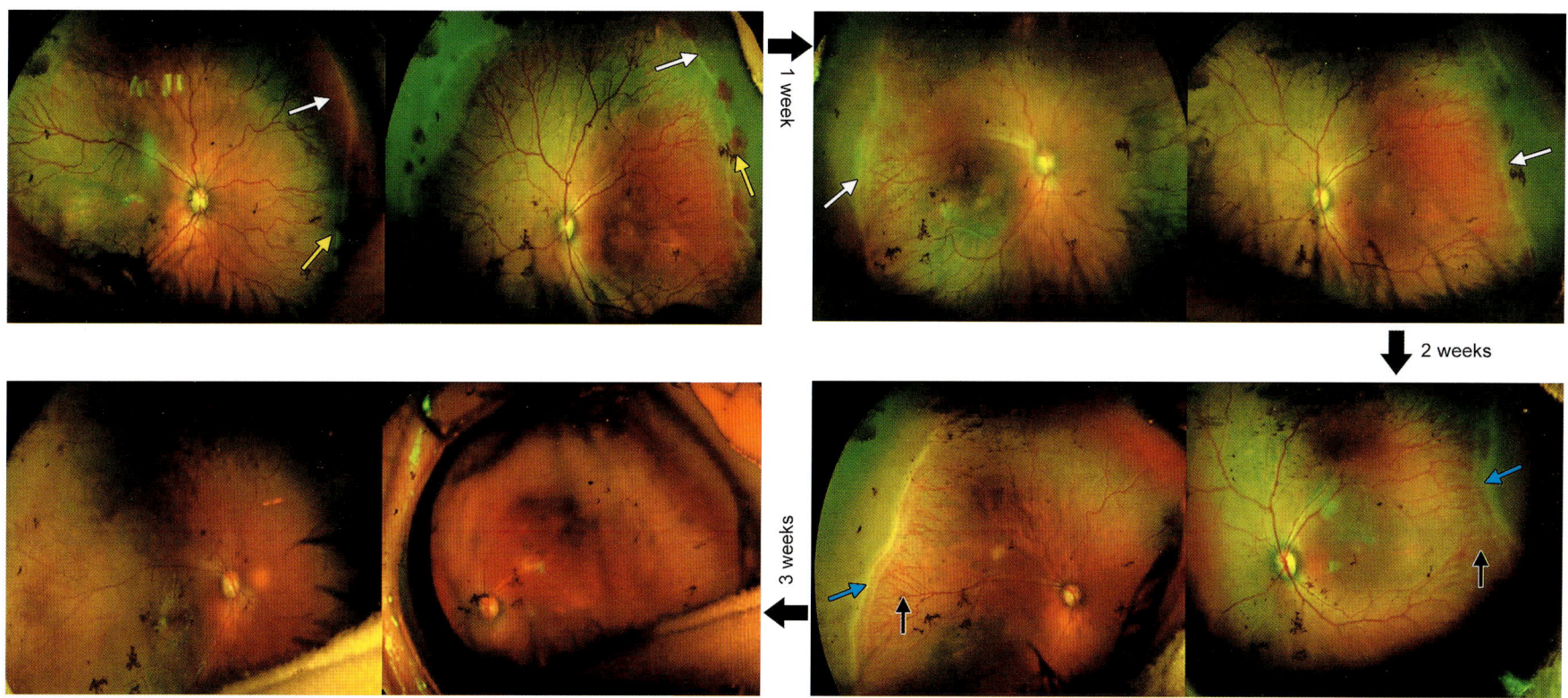

Fig. 17: UWF fundus images of OU of a 32 weeks PMA baby with a 28 weeks GA and 990 g BW with stage 2 flat ridge (white arrow), flat hemorrhages (yellow arrow), and preplus (upper right panel) showing signs of regression like resolved hemorrhages in 1 week follow-up (upper left panel). Ridge doubling (blue arrows) and peripheral vessel straightening (black arrows) can be seen in further 2 weeks follow-up (bottom left panel). Disappearance of ridge with regressed vessel tortuosity can be seen on further a 3 weeks follow-up (bottom right panel) without any form of intervention. (BW: birth weight; GA: gestational age; OU: both eyes; PMA: postmenstrual age; UWF: ultra-wide field)

REFERENCES

1. Jalali S, Azad R, Trehan HS, Trehan HS, Dogra MR, Gopal L, et al. Technical aspects of laser treatment for acute retinopathy of prematurity under topical anesthesia. Indian J Ophthalmol. 2010;58(6):509-15.
2. Lira RP, Calheiros AB, Barbosa MM, Barbosa MMM, Oliveira CV, Viana SL, et al. Efficacy and safety of green laser photocoagulation for threshold retinopathy of prematurity. Arq Bras Oftalmol. 2008;71(1):49-51.
3. Mintz-Hittner HA, Kennedy KA, Chuang AZ; BEAT-ROP Cooperative Group. Efficacy of intravitreal bevacizumab for stage 3+ retinopathy of prematurity. N Engl J Med. 2011;364(7):603-15.
4. Wallace DK, Dean TW, Hartnett ME, Kong L, Smith LE, Hubbard GB, et al. A dosing study of bevacizumab for retinopathy of prematurity: Late Recurrences and additional treatments. Ophthalmology. 2018;125(12):1961-6.
5. Roohipoor R, Karkhaneh R, Riazi-Esfahani M, Ghasemi F, Nili-Ahmadabadi M. Surgical management in advanced stages of retinopathy of prematurity; our experience. J Ophthalmic Vis Res. 2009;4(3):185-190.
6. Agarwal K, Jayanna S, Jalali S. Surgical management of retinopathy of prematurity. In: Cutting-edge vitreoretinal Surgery. Singapore: Springer; 2021. pp. 399-410.

CHAPTER 6

Uncommon Associations in Retinopathy of Prematurity

■ INTRODUCTION

This chapter is focused on uncommon associated pathologies which can coexist with ROP, which in turn underscores the importance of a multidisciplinary and a holistic approach to the eye care of premature infants.

■ BOTH EYES IMMATURE ZONE III WITH DISC ANOMALY

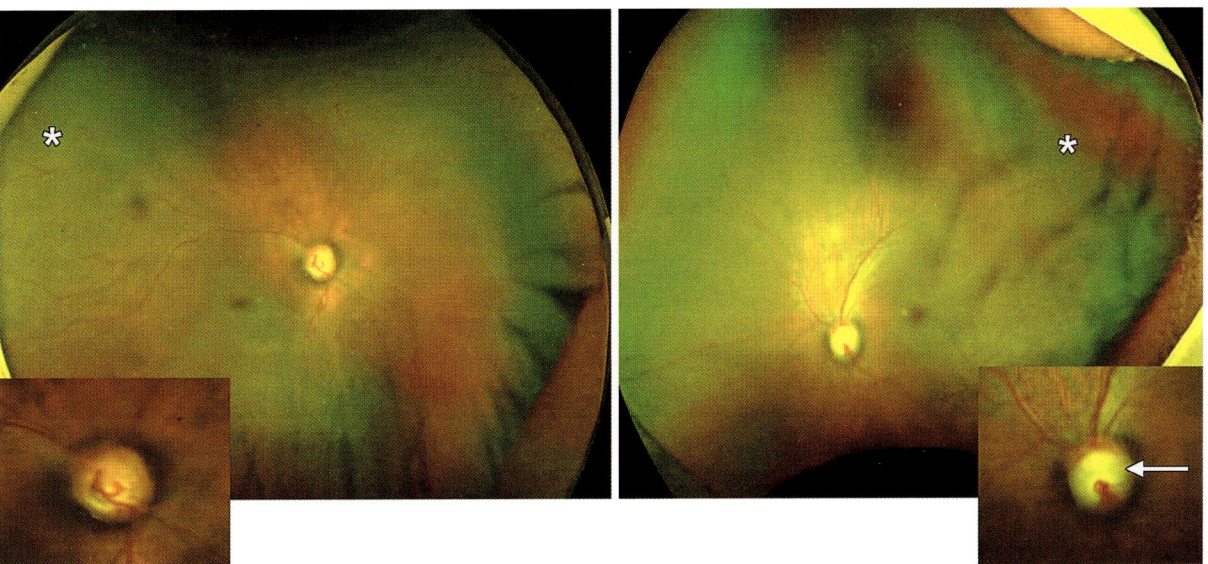

Fig. 1: OU UWF fundus photos of baby with 39 weeks PMA, 33 weeks GA and 1,700 g BW.

Note: Zone III immature retina (asterisks) showing congenital disc anomaly probably optic disc pit (white arrow in the inset images).
(BW: birth weight; GA: gestational age; OU: both eyes; PMA: postmenstrual age; UWF: ultra-wide field)

■ LEFT EYE STAGE 2, ZONE II, PREPLUS WITH VASCULAR ANOMOLY AT DISC

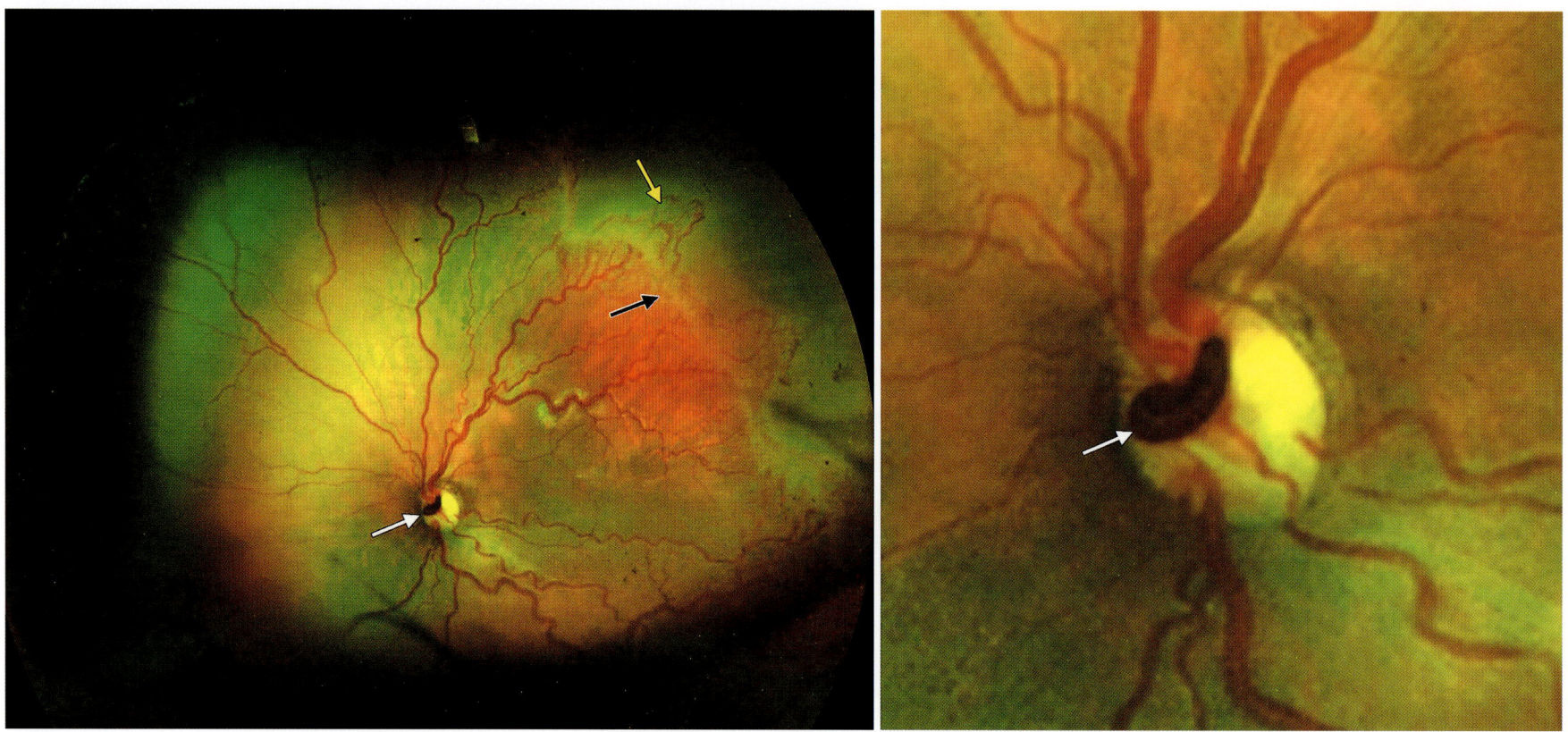

Fig. 2: OS UWF fundus photos of baby with 38 week PMA, 34 weeks GA and 2,000 g BW. The baby has stage 2 flat ridge (black arrow) in zone II preplus tortuosity of vessels along with vessel looping beyond the ridge (yellow arrow).

Note: Vascular anomaly at disc (white arrow) in the magnified image of disc (right).
(BW: birth weight; GA: gestational age; OS: left eye; PMA: postmenstrual age; UWF: ultra-wide field)

LEFT EYE ZONE II AVASCULAR PREPLUS WITH DISC HEMORRHAGE DUE TO PROBABLE POSTERIOR PERSISTENT FETAL VASCULATURE

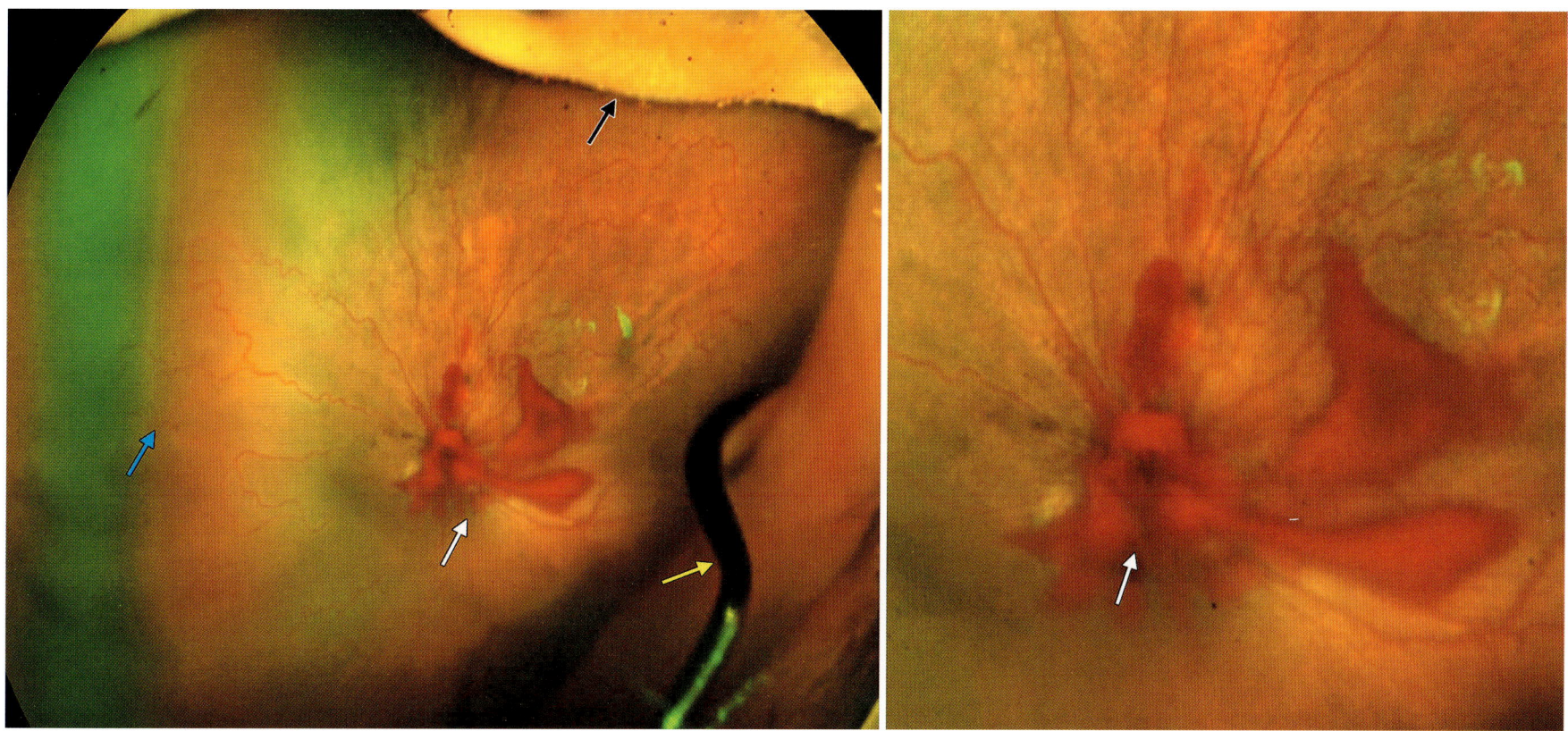

Fig. 3: OS UWF fundus photos of baby with 34 weeks PMA, 28 weeks GA and 1,000 g BW. The baby had looping of blood vessels (blue arrow), preplus vessel tortuosity in zone II, and hemorrhage at the disc (white arrow) obscuring it, probably secondary to posterior persistent fetal vasculature (right magnified view). Nose artifact (black arrow) and speculum artifact (yellow arrow) can be seen. (BW: birth weight; GA: gestational age; OS: left eye; PMA: postmenstrual age; UWF: ultra-wide field)

■ RIGHT EYE ZONE II, STAGE 3 PREPLUS WITH TORPEDO LESION TEMPORAL TO FOVEA

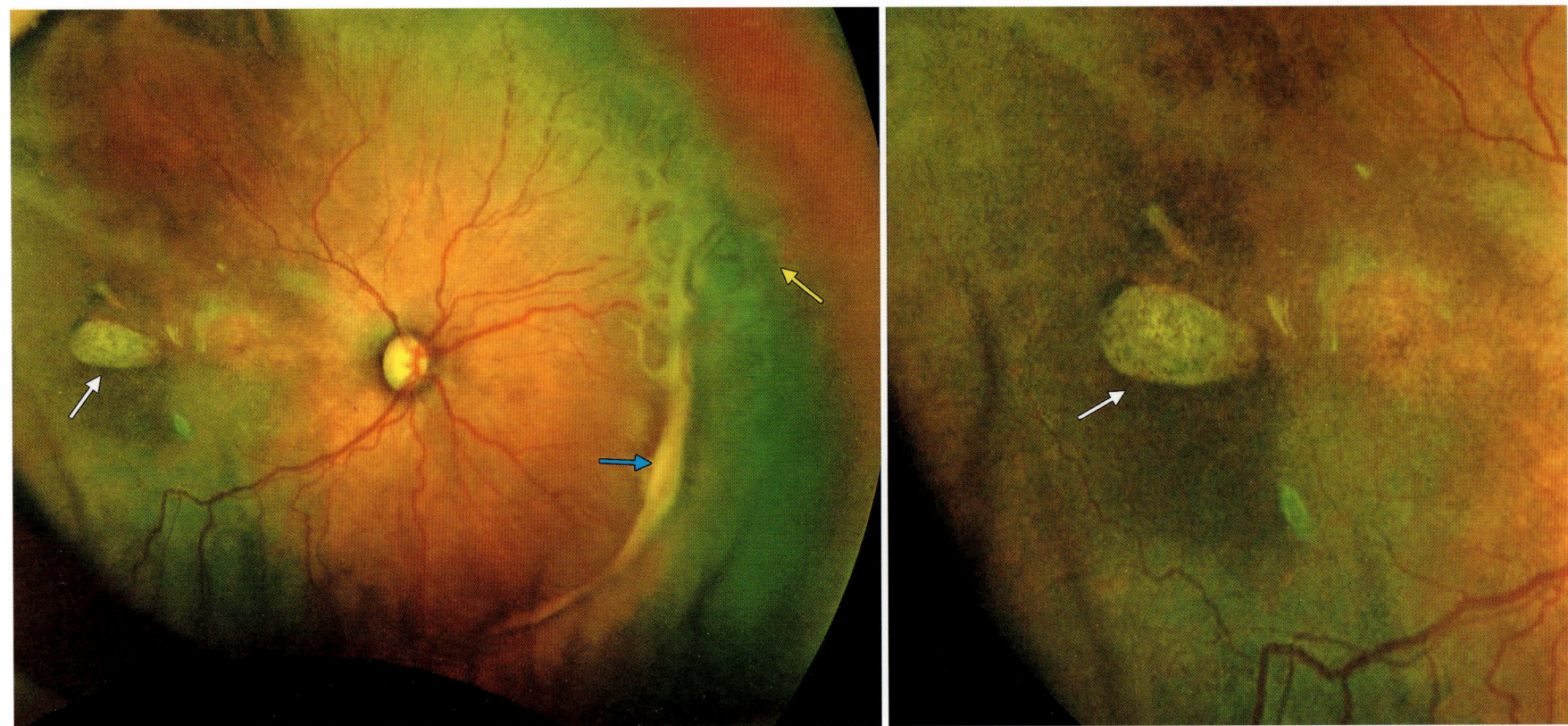

Fig. 4: OD UWF fundus photos of baby with 36 weeks PMA, 28 weeks GA and 1,100 g BW with preplus tortuosity of vessels, elevated ridge (blue arrow) in zone II, and flat retina beyond the ridge (yellow arrow).

Note: The torpedo-shaped chorioretinal atrophic patch temporal to fovea (white arrow) with tip pointing toward fovea (right magnified view).
(BW: birth weight; GA: gestational age; OD: right eye; PMA: postmenstrual age; UWF: ultra-wide field)

■ BOTH EYES IMMATURE ZONE III IN LIGHTLY PIGMENTED FUNDUS

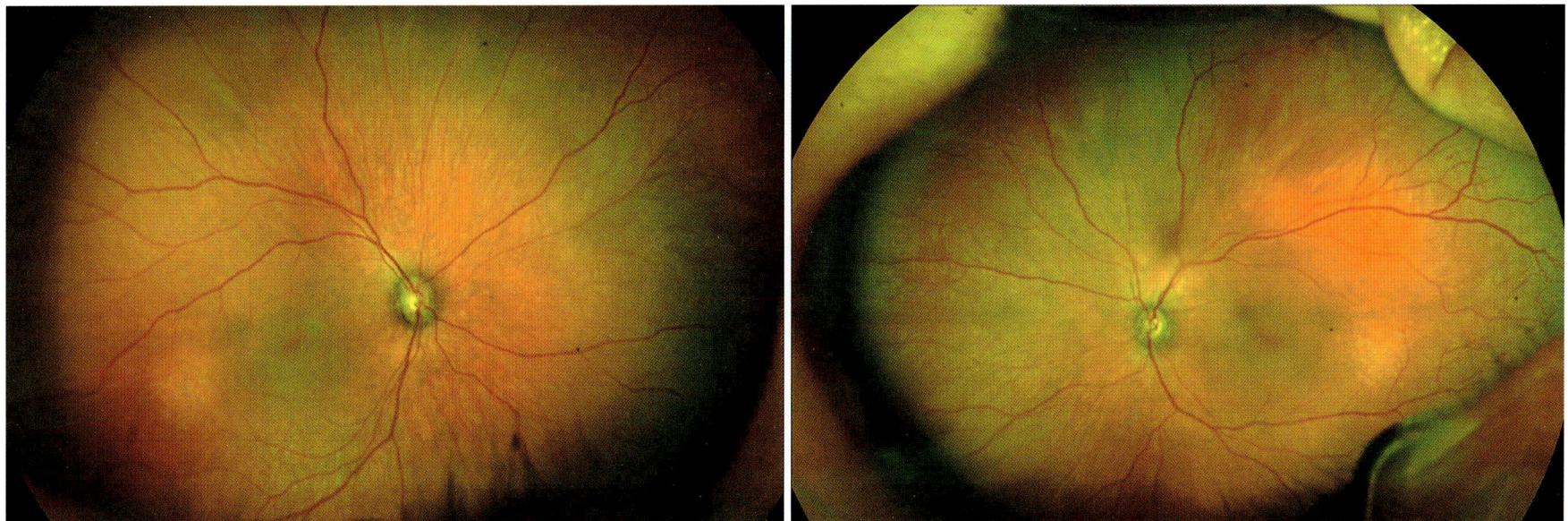

Fig. 5: OU UWF fundus photos of baby with 39 weeks PMA, 32 weeks GA and 1,000 g BW.

Note: Immature vessels in zone III in lightly pigmented fundi.
(BW: birth weight; GA: gestational age; OU: both eyes; PMA: postmenstrual age; UWF: ultra-wide field)

EPIRETINAL MEMBRANE SECONDARY TO LASER IN EYE PRETREATED WITH BEVACIZUMAB

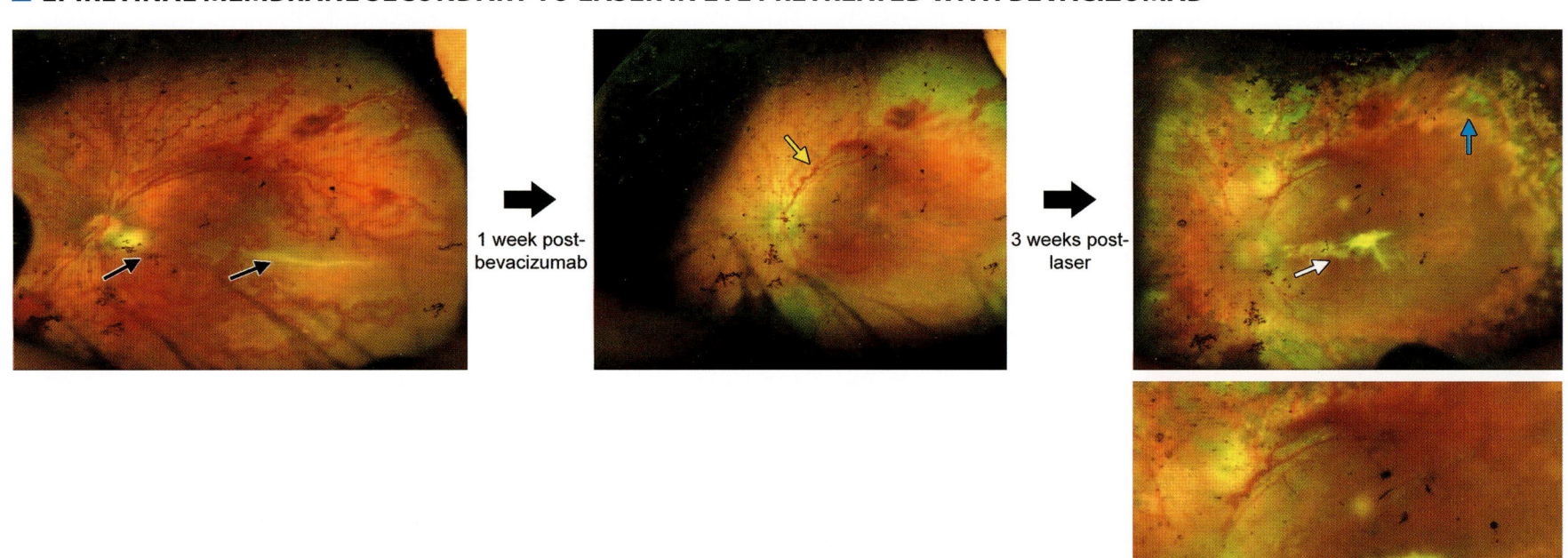

Fig. 6: OS 34 weeks PMA baby with 28 weeks GA and 1,200 g BW. The baby had A-ROP (top left) and exudation (black arrow) in the posterior pole. 1 week after the intravitreal bevacizumab, the vessel tortuosity reduced, but not completely gone (top center). A complete regression occurred 3 weeks after the additional retinal lasers (top right). Adequate laser marks (blue arrow) in periphery and epiretinal membrane (white arrow) at fovea are seen (top right). Magnified image of epiretinal membrane is seen in the bottom right image (white arrow). (BW: birth weight; GA: gestational age; OS: left eye; PMA: postmenstrual age; UWF: ultra-wide field)

CHAPTER 7: Artifact in Ultra-Wide Field Photos

INTRODUCTION

Inevitably, any imaging modality carries associated artifacts, which one needs to be aware of to prevent misinterpretation, especially in unforgiving conditions like retinopathy of prematurity. This chapter highlights several common artifacts in ultra-wide field color fundus imaging, apart from the notable limitation of false red-green images encountered with the Optos fundus camera.

COMMON ARTIFACTS ON OPTOS IMAGES

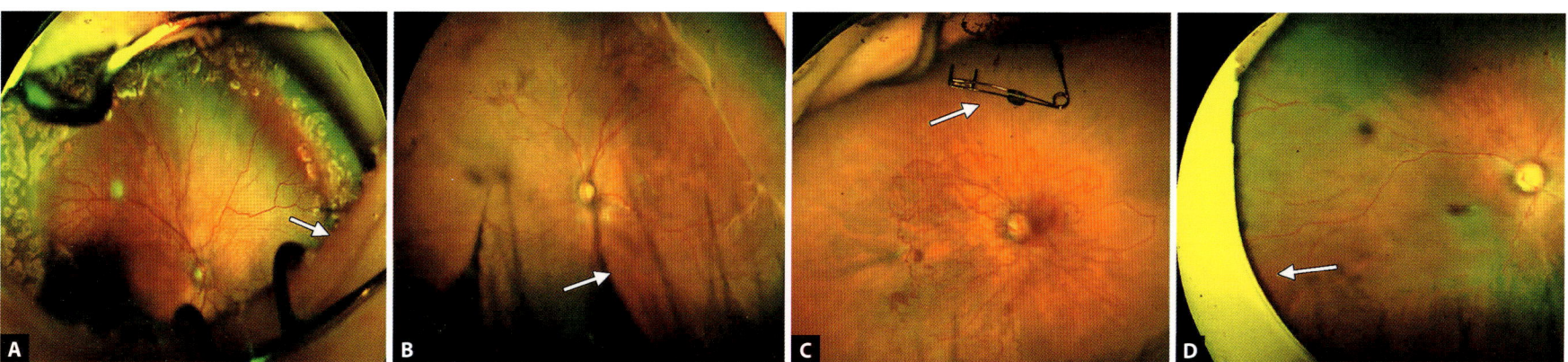

Figs. 1A to D: (A) Speculum and eye lids artifact (white arrow); (B) Eye lash artifact (white arrow); (C) Speculum artifact (white arrow); (D) Camera aperture margin artifact (white arrow).

■ SHADOW ARTIFACTS BLOCKING POSTERIOR POLE AND HORIZONTAL QUADRANTS OF IMAGES

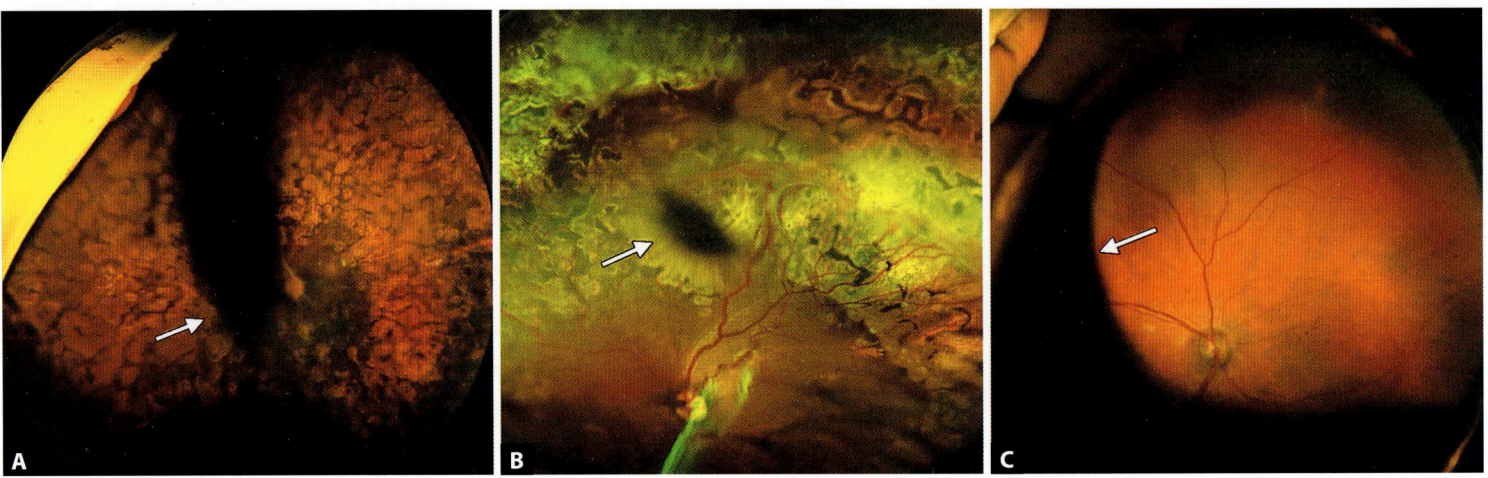

Figs. 2A to C: (A) Shadow artifact due to finger (white arrow); (B) Shadow artifact due to persistent anterior fetal vasculature (white arrow); (C) Shadow artifact due to improper eye alignment (white arrow).

■ NOSE ARTIFACTS

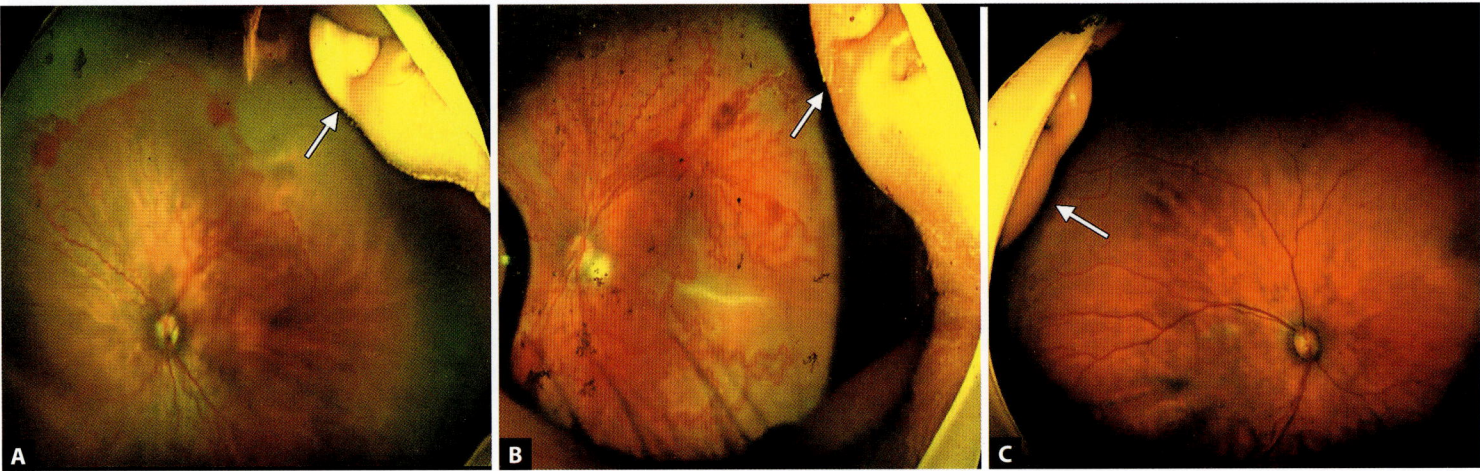

Figs. 3A to C: Various ultra-wide field photos showing nose artifacts covering superotemporal quadrants (white arrows).

■ REFLECTION ARTIFACTS

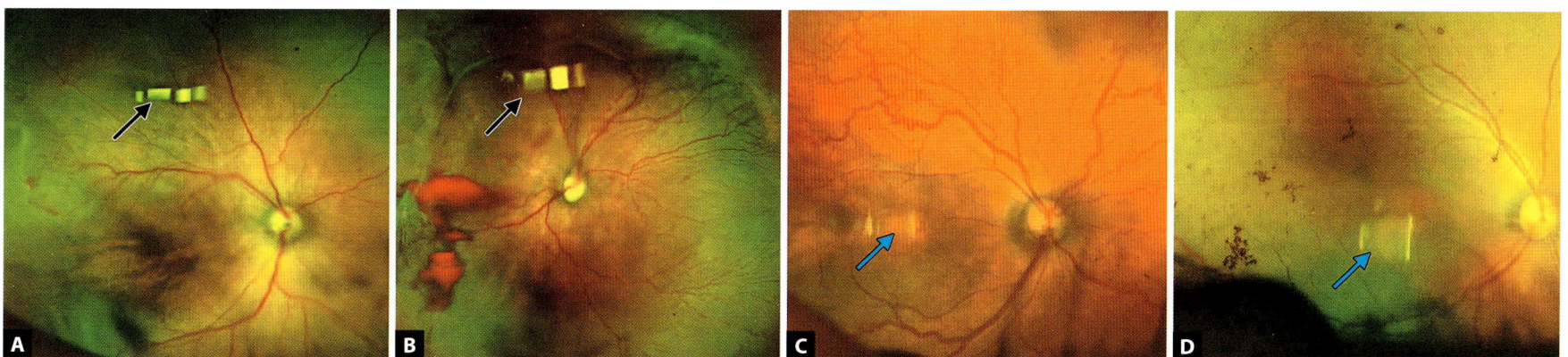

Figs. 4A to D: Various ultra-wide field photos showing reflection artifacts commonly seen in posterior pole (blue arrows) and superior quadrants (black arrows).

■ ARTIFACTS DUE TO VITREOUS CONTENTS

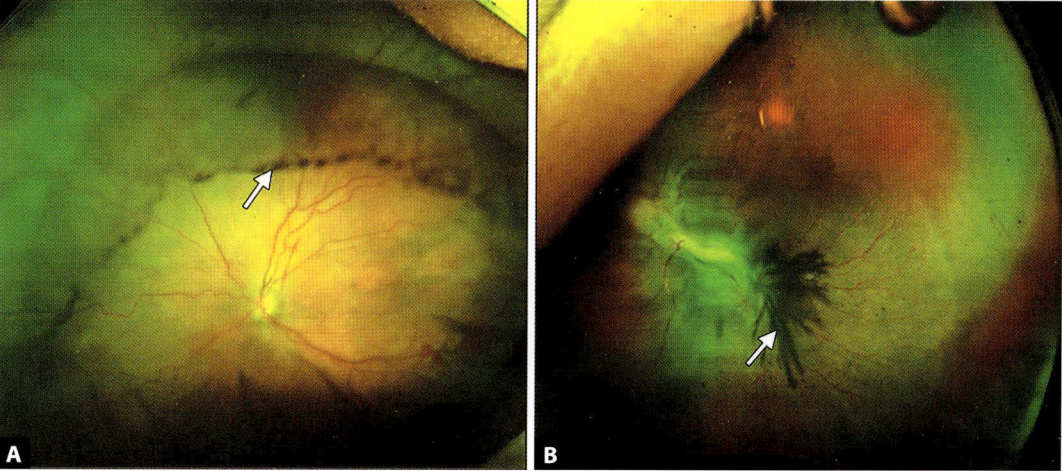

Figs. 5A and B: (A) Opacity due to vitreous hemorrhage (white arrow); (B) Opacity due to anterior fetal vasculature behind lens (white arrow).

Index

Page numbers followed by *f* refer to figure.

A

Anterior fetal vasculature 66*f*, 67*f*
Antivascular endothelial growth factor therapy 39
Aperture artifact 12*f*
Avascular retina 8*f*
Avascular zone, persistence of 48*f*

B

Bevacizumab 39, 64
Birth weight 41*f*, 46, 47, 49, 53, 54, 56, 59, 60, 62, 63
B-scan 46

C

Congenital disc anomaly 59
Cycloplegics 46

D

Diffuse exudative detachment 46
Disc hemorrhage 61

E

Elevated retina 45*f*
Epiretinal membrane 53, 64, 64*f*
    magnified image of 64*f*
Extensive avascular retina 21*f*
Extensive laser 46
    photocoagulation treatment 37
Extensive preretinal hemorrhage 20*f*
Extensive tortuous vessels 54
Exudation 53, 54

F

Exudative detachment 38, 38*f*, 54
Eye
    care 59
    lids artifact 65*f*
Eyelash artefacts 18*f*, 30*f*, 47, 65*f*

F

Fibrovascular proliferation 33
Flat hemorrhages 13*f*, 17*f*
Flat retina 27
Flying baby
    positioning, modified 2
    technique, modified 3
Fovea 19*f*, 20*f*, 21*f*, 32, 34

G

Gestational age 5, 5*f*, 41*f*, 46, 47, 49, 53, 54, 56, 59, 60, 62, 63

H

Holistic approach 59
Hot dog-like linear
    hemorrhage 22, 24, 56
    red lesions 22
Human fetal retinal vascularization 35
Hybrid retinopathy of prematurity 35

I

Immature retina 6
Immature vessels 63

I

Improper eye alignment 66*f*
Inferonasal quadrant 17*f*
International Classification of Retinopathy of Prematurity 9, 22
Intravitreal antivascular endothelial growth factor 34, 39
Intravitreal bevacizumab 47-53, 64*f*
Irreversible blindness 7

L

Laser
    photocoagulation 34, 36*f*, 39, 42*f*, 53, 54
    treatment 43*f*

M

Macula 34
Mature retina 5
Modified flying baby positioning 3*f*

N

Nasal retina 33
Neonatal endophthalmitis 37
Nose artifacts 66, 66*f*
Notch sign 22, 29*f*

O

Opacity 67*f*
Optic disc pit 59
Optimal positioning of eye 3*f*

Optos
    fundus camera 65
    modification to existing apertures of 4

P

Panretinal laser photocoagulation 8*f*
Pars plana vitrectomy 40, 55, 55*f*
Peripheral vessel straightening 57*f*
Plus and preplus disease 11
Popcorn lesions 23, 25*f*-27*f*
Posterior elevated ridge 27*f*
Posterior flat ridge 27*f*
Posterior persistent fetal vasculature 61
Posterior pole 67*f*
    vasculature, severe tortuosity of 8*f*
    vessel 13*f*
        persistence of 49
        tortuosity 15*f*
Posterior ridge elevation 26*f*
Postmenstrual age 5*f*, 28*f*, 41*f*, 46, 47, 49, 53, 54, 55*f*, 56, 59, 60, 62, 63
Preplus vessel tortuosity 61*f*
Preretinal hemorrhage 8*f*, 18, 18*f*, 19, 19*f*, 20, 31, 45, 47, 49, 53, 55*f*
Pupils 3*f*

R

Ranibizumab 39
Reflection artefact 5*f*, 13*f*, 15*f*, 42*f*, 67, 67*f*
Regression, signs of 39
Removable camera aperture 4*f*
Retina 5
Retinal detachment 19*f*, 46
Retinal edema 37
Retinal vascular changes 11
Retinal vascularization 5
Retinal vessels 5*f*, 17*f*, 25*f*
Retinal zones 10
Retinopathy of prematurity 1, 7-9, 21, 22, 33-37, 39, 51, 56, 57, 59
    aggressive 7, 38, 41*f*, 49, 50, 53, 54
    half zone 34
    regressing aggressive 47, 52-54
    spontaneous regression of 22
    surgery in 40
    visualize 34
Rhegmatogenous detachment 40
Ridge doubling 22, 27*f*, 56

S

Severe dilatation 17*f*
Speculum 65*f*
    artifact 15*f*, 61*f*, 65*f*
Sterile speculum 3*f*
Superior quadrants 67*f*
Superotemporal quadrant 29*f*, 66*f*

T

Temporal linear hemorrhage 24*f*
Temporal notch 29*f*
Thrombocytopenia 31
Topical anesthesia 3*f*
Topical steroids 46
Torpedo-shaped chorioretinal atrophic patch 62
Tortuous peripheral vessels 14*f*
Tortuous posterior vessels 14*f*
Tortuous vessels 17*f*, 29*f*
Total avascular retina 17*f*
Trauma, birth related 30

U

Ultra-wide field 33*f*, 41*f*, 46, 47, 49, 53, 54, 56, 59, 60, 62, 63
    fundus
        images 1, 5*f*, 8*f*, 11, 12*f*, 13*f*, 15*f*-19*f*, 21*f*, 23*f*-33*f*, 35*f*, 37*f*, 41*f*-55*f*, 56, 57*f*, 59*f*, 60, 61*f*, 63*f*, 66*f*, 67*f*
        imaging technique 1

V

Vascular anomaly 60
Vascular retina 13*f*
Vessels 15*f*
    looping of 8*f*
    mild tortuosity of 11*f*, 26*f*, 27*f*, 29*f*, 56
    persistent tortuosity of 45*f*
    preplus tortuosity of 60*f*, 62*f*
    reduced tortuosity of 47
    regressed tortuosity of 46
Viral retinitis 37
Visual feedback monitor 4*f*
Vitreous hemorrhage 19*f*, 30, 45*f*, 67*f*